组织胚胎实验学

（双语版）

黄少萍　主编

东南大学出版社
SOUTHEAST UNIVERSITY PRESS
·南京·

内 容 简 介

本书由中英文对照的组织学、胚胎学总论、彩图组成。全书共19章实验内容，1—17章为组织学，18—19章为胚胎学总论。各章节有实验目的、实验内容、思考题三部分。在实验内容中，从肉眼、低倍、高倍指导学生循序渐进地观察结构，培养学生观察切片的能力。全书有96张彩图，附英文标注。胚胎学总论的彩图来自学生上课用的模型。

本书适用普通高等医学院校、药学院校等8年制、7年制、5年制临床医学及相关专业学生、医学留学生等使用。

图书在版编目(CIP)数据

组织胚胎实验学：双语版：汉英对照/黄少萍主编.
—南京：东南大学出版社，2019.7
ISBN 978-7-5641-8450-6

Ⅰ.①组… Ⅱ.①黄… Ⅲ.①人体组织学—人体胚胎学—实验—双语教学—教材—汉、英 Ⅳ.①R329.1-33

中国版本图书馆CIP数据核字(2019)第123773号

组织胚胎实验学(双语版)

主　　编　黄少萍
出版发行　东南大学出版社
出 版 人　江建中
责任编辑　陈　淑
社　　址　南京市四牌楼2号　(邮编:210096)

经　　销　全国各地新华书店
印　　刷　江苏凤凰数码印务有限公司
开　　本　787 mm×1092 mm　1/16
印　　张　7
彩　　页　16页
字　　数　188千
版　　次　2019年7月第1版
印　　次　2019年7月第1次印刷
书　　号　ISBN　978-7-5641-8450-6
定　　价　30.00元

(本社图书若有印装质量问题，请直接与营销部联系。电话(传真)：025—83791830)

《组织胚胎实验学》
编　委　会

主　编　黄少萍

副主编　夏江燕　吴晓菁　张昕昕

编　委

吴晓菁（东南大学）　　张昕昕（东南大学）

朱丽娟（东南大学）　　李　娜（东南大学）

沈　杨（东南大学）　　陆　静（东南大学）

夏江燕（东南大学）　　黄少萍（东南大学）

纪　红（江苏省肿瘤医院）　　杨　宁（东南大学）

徐淑芬（东南大学）　　毛　曦（东南大学）

卢　莹（南京医科大学附属妇产医院）

李苏影（南京医科大学第二附属医院）

前言

实验课是教学过程的重要环节，是理论教学的有效补充。通过实验教学，学生能够理论联系实际，提高分析问题、解决问题的能力。为了适应21世纪人才培养和双语教学的需求，我们在原教研室杨宁主任（主编）和其他主编、编委所编写的《组织胚胎实验学》的基础上，结合实验室的切片，编写了《组织胚胎实验学》（双语版）。

在各位编委的共同努力下，《组织胚胎实验学》（双语版）顺利完成。本书包含组织学内容17章，胚胎学总论2章，彩图96张并附英文标注。书中各章中、英文相间排版，方便8年制临床医学全英班和留学生学习。同时，结合理论教学要求，每个章节包含实验目的、实验内容、思考题三部分。对每张切片，按照由肉眼—低倍—高倍循序渐进的原则，指导学生有序观察，并标明观察要点，引导学生观察重点结构。

本教材依托于前版教材良好的基础，在此，谨向原教研室杨宁副教授（主编）、徐淑芬副教授、毛曦副教授，以及其他主编、编委表示深深的敬意和感谢！

由于编者水平有限，如有错误和不妥之处，恳请同行专家和读者给予批评和指教！

东南大学　黄少萍

前言

目 录

Contents

第一章
绪　　论

一、实验目的

1. 掌握组织学石蜡切片的制备过程。

2. 掌握 HE 染色步骤以及嗜酸性、嗜碱性的含义。

二、实验内容

1. 石蜡切片的制备

（1）取材：冰上操作，新鲜的动物或人体组织，切成约 0.5～1 cm^3 小块。

（2）固定：用 4%的多聚甲醛液或 75%乙醇，室温固定 12～24 h。

（3）脱水：固定好的组织块含有水分，组织一般放置于浓度逐级递升的乙醇（70%→80%→90%→100%）中，各放置数小时，进行脱水。随后组织放入二甲苯，置换出组织中的乙醇，使其透明。

（4）包埋：经过透明的组织浸入融化的石蜡液中 2 h 左右，再将组织移入盛有石蜡液的包埋框中，冷却即为石蜡标本。

（5）切片：蜡块固定在石蜡切片机上，切成 5～8 μm 的薄片，在 42 ℃水中展片，随后平贴在载玻片上，烘干备用。

2. HE 染色

（1）水化：石蜡切片用二甲苯脱蜡约 30 min，随后在浓度逐级递降的乙醇（100%→90%→80%→70%）内，各放置数分钟，然后于蒸馏水中放置数分钟。

（2）染色：苏木精为碱性染料，可将细胞核染成蓝色；伊红为酸性染料，可将细胞质染成红色。经染色的切片，再经过逐级递升的乙醇脱水、二甲苯透明，随后在组织上滴加树胶，加盖玻片封存。

三、思考题

1. 简述石蜡切片的制备过程。

2. 什么是嗜酸性？什么是嗜碱性？

（黄少萍，李娜）

Chapter 1
Introduction

Ⅰ. Experiment purpose

1. To master the preparation process of histological paraffin sections.
2. Grasp the steps of HE staining and the meaning of eosinophilic and basophilic.

Ⅱ. Experiment contents

1. Preparation of paraffin sections

(1) Materials: This part is operated on ice. Animal or human tissue is cut into about 0.5-1 cm^3.

(2) Fixation: The tissue block is fixed with 4% paraformaldehyde or 75% ethanol at room temperature for 12-24 h.

(3) Dehydration: The fixed tissue block contains water, and the tissue is processed with step-up alcohol (70% → 80% → 90% → 100%) (each for several hours) for dehydration. The tissue is then treated with xylene for replacing alcohol from the tissue to make it transparent.

(4) Embedding: Tissue is immersed in paraffin solution for about 2 h, then tissue is transferred into the embedding frame containing paraffin solution until the paraffin sample is cooled.

(5) Slice: The wax block is fixed on the paraffin slicer and cut into 5-8 μm thin slices, which are spread in 42 ℃ water, then flat on the slide and dried for later use.

2. HE staining

(1) Hydration: Paraffin sections are dewaxed with xylene for about 30 min, followed by each several minutes of progressively decreasing alcohol (100%→90%→80%→70%), and then the paraffin sections are placed in distilled water for several

minutes.

(2) Staining: Hematoxylin is an alkaline dye, which can dyes the nucleus blue. Eosin is an acid dye that stains the cytoplasm red. The stained sections are dehydrated with step by step alcohol and transparent with xylene. Then resin is added on the tissue and sealed with cover glass.

III. Questions

1. Briefly describe the preparation process of paraffin section.
2. What is eosinophilic? What is basophilic?

(Huang Shaoping, Li Na)

第二章
上 皮 组 织

一、实验目的

1. 掌握上皮组织的一般特征与分类。
2. 掌握各种被覆上皮的光镜结构特点及分布。
3. 掌握上皮组织的特殊结构特点与作用。

二、实验内容

1. 单层扁平上皮（Simple squamous epithelium）（彩图 1）

（1）取材和染色：小肠，HE 染色。

（2）观察：

肉眼：可见红色、圆形的中空组织，为小肠的横断面。其外表面被覆的单层扁平上皮为间皮。

低倍：小肠管壁的外表面被覆单层扁平上皮，为间皮；另，管壁中找到小血管横断面，内含有红细胞，其腔面衬贴的单层扁平上皮为内皮。

高倍：细胞呈扁平状，含细胞核处切面略厚，核略向腔内突出，染成紫蓝色；无核处胞质很薄，呈细线状。

（3）观察要点：肠管外表面、血管内表面的单层扁平上皮。

2. 单层立方上皮（Simple cuboidal epithelium）（彩图 2）

（1）取材和染色：甲状腺，HE 染色。

（2）观察：

肉眼：可见一淡紫红色的组织。

低倍：镜下可见大小不等的甲状腺滤泡，呈圆形或椭圆形。滤泡壁由单层立方上皮围成，腔内有均质状粉红色的胶质。

高倍：上皮细胞为立方形，单层排列，核圆形，位于细胞中央，胞质嗜酸性。

（3）观察要点：滤泡上皮细胞的形态。

3. 单层柱状上皮（Simple columnar epithelium）（彩图 3）

（1）取材和染色：小肠，HE 染色。

（2）观察：

肉眼：腔面几个大突起为皱襞，其表面有许多小突起，为小肠绒毛。

低倍：找到皱襞及小肠绒毛，其表面被覆的是单层柱状上皮。

高倍：上皮细胞为柱状，核呈椭圆形，近细胞基底部，细胞游离面可见薄层淡红色的纹状缘（即电镜下观察到的微绒毛）。柱状细胞间可见杯状细胞，形似高脚酒杯，核染色深，呈三角形或半月形，靠近细胞基部，顶部胞质充满粘原颗粒，制片过程中溶解后，胞质呈空泡状。

（3）观察要点：柱状上皮细胞及纹状缘、杯状细胞。

4. 假复层纤毛柱状上皮（Pseudostratified ciliated columnar epithelium）（彩图 4）

（1）取材和染色：气管，HE 染色。

（2）观察：

肉眼：气管壁中可见"C"形蓝色的透明软骨环，腔面被覆有薄层深染的假复层纤毛柱状上皮。

低倍：分清蓝色的透明软骨，找到腔面被覆的假复层纤毛柱状上皮。上皮细胞核位置高低不齐，似复层，细胞间夹有杯状细胞。

高倍：上皮由柱状细胞、杯状细胞、梭形细胞和锥体细胞组成。细胞基部均附着在基膜上，故上皮为单层。柱状细胞呈柱状，核位置较高，游离面可见纤毛，胞质嗜酸性。梭形细胞核居细胞中部，锥体细胞核呈圆形靠近基膜。上皮基膜较明显。杯状细胞形态见"单层柱状上皮"中所述。

（3）观察要点：柱状细胞及其纤毛、杯状细胞、基膜等。

5. 复层扁平上皮（Stratified squamous epithelium）（彩图 5）

（1）取材和染色：食管，HE 染色。

（2）观察：

肉眼：食管腔面凹凸不平，腔面被覆一层紫蓝色的复层扁平上皮（未角化）。上皮下方为淡红色的结缔组织和深红色的肌组织。

低倍：上皮细胞排列紧密，有多层，从基底部至表层细胞染色逐渐变浅。上皮组织基底面呈波浪状，表面无角化层。

高倍：上皮细胞形态不一，基底部为一层立方形或矮柱状细胞，附着在基膜上，染色较深，核呈椭圆形。中间数层为多边形细胞，细胞较大，核呈圆形或椭圆形，表面几层为扁平或扁梭形细胞，染色较浅，核呈梭形。

(3) 观察要点:上皮各层细胞的形态变化。

6. 变移上皮 (Transitional epithelium)(彩图 6)

(1) 取材和染色:膀胱(收缩状态),HE 染色。

(2) 观察:

肉眼:膀胱腔面可见紫蓝色一层,为变移上皮,因膀胱收缩而呈现凹凸不平。

低倍:上皮细胞层次较多,基底部的细胞小,表层细胞较大。

高倍:表层细胞为大立方形,核 1～2 个;中间数层为多边形的细胞,基底层细胞呈低柱状或立方形,细胞体积小。当膀胱充盈时,细胞层次减少,上皮厚度变薄,细胞形状变扁。

(3) 观察要点:各层细胞的形态变化。

三、思考题

1. 上皮组织的一般特征是什么?上皮组织分几种类型?被覆上皮的分类依据是什么?

2. 复层扁平上皮和变移上皮的光镜特点有何不同?

3. 单层扁平上皮主要分布在哪里?

(李娜,黄少萍)

Chapter 2
Epithelial Tissue

Ⅰ. Experiment purpose

1. To master the general characteristic and types of epithelial tissue.

2. To master the structure features of every kind of covering epithelia under light microscope and their distribution.

3. To master the special construction features and action of epithelial tissue.

Ⅱ. Experiment contents

1. Simple squamous epithelium (Fig. 1)

(1) Material and staining: Appendix, HE staining.

(2) Observe:

By eyes: A round pink hollow organ, is the transverse cutting of the small intestine. A simple squamous epithelium covers the outer surface of the small intestine wall (mesothelium).

Lower power lens: The wall of small intestine contains smooth muscle stained red, and its outer surface is covered by the mesothelium. In the wall of the small intestine, there are some small blood vessels containing some red blood cells. The inner surface of vessels is covered by endothelium(simple squamous epithelium).

Higher power lens: Mesothelial cells were flat, the cytoplasm lacking the nuclear site is very thin, and the nuclear dyed into blue slightly protrudes into the lumen.

(3) Observation key points: Mesothelium and endothelium.

2. Simple cuboidal epithelium (Fig. 2)

(1) Material and staining: Thyroid, HE staining.

(2) Observe:

By eyes: The tissue is stained in red or amaranth.

Lower power lens: The tissue contains many round or oval follicles which are different in volum. The wall of the follicles is consisted of a single layer of simple cuboidal epithelium. The lumen contains the colloid which is stained in red color.

Higher power lens: The cuboidal cells are arranged in one layer, the cell boundaries more clearly and cytoplasm is acidophilic, the nuclear locates in the center of the cells.

(3) Observation key points: The structure of the cuboidal cells.

3. Simple columnar epithelium (Fig. 3)

(1) Material and staining: Small intestine, HE staining.

(2) Observe:

By eyes: In the surface of lumen, there are some large protrusions, known as the plica. At the plica surface there are some small protrusions, called villi coated by the simple columnar epithelium.

Lower power lens: Found the plica and the villi, obviously their surfaces are covered with simple columnar epithelium.

Higher power lens: Lateral view, the high columnar cells are closely arranged in one layer, their free surface of the epithelial cell contains a thin layer of brush border (when observed by the electron microscope, the brush border is consisted of microvilli). The cell boundaries more clearly and cytoplasm is stained in red, the nuclear is oval and locates near the base of the cells. Between the columnar cells, there are some goblet cell looked like a cup. In the upper part of the cell, the mucus granules are dissolved during the HE process, so the cytoplasm of goblet cell is hollow after HE staining.

(3) Observation key points: Columnar cell and its brush border.

4. Pseudostratified ciliated columnar epithelium (Fig. 4)

(1) Material and staining: Trachea, HE staining.

(2) Observe:

By eyes: A C-shaped blue hyaline cartilage ring can be seen in the wall of the trachea, and the lumen surface has a layer epithelial which is strongly stained in blue or bluish violet.

Lower power lens: The lumen surface is covered by pseudostratified ciliated columnar epithelium looked like several layers owing to different heights of different kinds of the cells. Between epithelial cells there are some goblet cells.

Higher power lens: The heights of different kinds of cells are different as if the epithelium contains several layers of cells. But all cells are based on the basement membrane, so the epithelium is the simple epithelium. Columnar cells have cilia in free surface. Nuclear of cone-shaped cell locates near to the basement membrane. Spindle cell's nuclear is located in the center part of cell. Goblet cell nucleus is also based on the bottom.

(3) Observation key points: Columnar cell and its cilia, goblet cell, basement membrane.

5. Stratified squamous epithelium (Fig. 5)

(1) Material and staining: Esophagus, HE staining.

(2) Observe:

By eyes: Lumen surface of esophagus is uneven, and the surface is covered by a thick layer of blue-violet epithelium (stratified squamous epithelium).

Lower power lens: Epithelial cells are closely arranged into several layers. From the basal layer to the apical part, the cells become a little light staining. The basal part of the epithelium is wavy and the lumen surface has no keratinized layer.

Higher power lens: Superficial several layers of cells are flat, which nucleus is the flat ellipse. Central several layers of cells are polygonal cells, whose nuclei are the circular located at the center. Base is a layer of low columnar or cubic cells. The boundary is unclear; the nucleus is round and stained in dark blue.

(3) Observation key points: Structure of different layers of the stratified squamous epithelium.

6. Transitional epithelium (Fig. 6)

(1) Material and Staining: Bladder (contraction), HE staining.

(2) Observe:

By eyes: Bladder's lumen surface is uneven and the indigo blue part is its internal surface.

Lower power lens: Epithelial tissue is closely arranged into several layers. The surface layer cell is big.

Higher power lens: The surface layer cells called domelike cells are big; the intermediate layer cells mostly are the polygon; the basal cells are cubic or low columnar. The amount of cell layers is increasing when bladder is empty. The layers of cells are reduced when bladder is ample.

(3) Observation key points: Structure of different layers of the transitional epithelium.

III. Questions

1. What are the general characteristics of epithelial tissue? How many types of

epithelium can be classified? Covering epithelia's classification is based on what?

2. How to distinguish the stratified squamous epithelium from the transitional epithelium under the light microscope?

3. Where are the distributions of the simple squamous epithelium?

(Li Na, Huang Shaoping)

第三章
结 缔 组 织

一、实验目的

1. 掌握结缔组织的一般特征与分类。

2. 掌握疏松结缔组织中的胶原纤维、弹性纤维、网状纤维、成纤维细胞、巨噬细胞、浆细胞和肥大细胞的光镜结构。

3. 熟悉致密结缔组织、脂肪组织和网状组织的结构特征。

二、实验内容

1. 疏松结缔组织铺片（Loose connective tissue stretched preparation）（彩图 7）

（1）取材和染色：小鼠肠系膜组织。取材前活体腹腔注射台盼蓝。取材、铺片与固定后，用苏木素、中性红和伊红等染色。

（2）观察：

肉眼：可见淡紫红色的染色组织。

低倍：镜下找到淡染区，可见纤维粗细不等，纵横交错，排列疏松。浅粉红色条带状的纤维为胶原纤维，蓝紫色的细而分支的纤维为弹性纤维。纤维之间分布有许多细胞，大多数细胞为成纤维细胞，胞质因染色浅淡不易观察，可见长椭圆形的成纤维细胞核。还可见散在分布的巨噬细胞（胞质含有蓝色的吞噬颗粒）。

高倍：镜下重点观察两种纤维和两种细胞的形态结构。

① 胶原纤维：数量较多，粗细不等，分支交错，排列疏松，染成粉红色。

② 弹性纤维：细而有分支，末端弯曲，有折光性，染成蓝紫色。

③ 成纤维细胞：数量最多，扁平多突起，细胞轮廓界限不太清楚，核大而呈卵圆形，浅染，胞质弱嗜碱性。

④ 巨噬细胞：大而不规则，核小深染，胞质嗜酸性，内含蓝紫色的吞噬颗粒。

（3）观察要点：胶原纤维、弹性纤维、成纤维细胞、巨噬细胞。

2. 疏松结缔组织、致密结缔组织和脂肪组织(Loose connective tissue, dense connective tissue and adipose tissue)(彩图 8)

(1) 取材和染色:手掌或足底皮肤,HE 染色。

(2) 观察:

肉眼:表面紫蓝色薄层为表皮。其下方红色部分为真皮,再下方浅染部分为皮下组织(疏松结缔组织和脂肪组织)。

低倍:真皮为致密结缔组织,染色较深(红色),向深部移动,染色较浅的部分为疏松结缔组织和脂肪组织。

高倍:在真皮处,可见粗大的胶原纤维束交错致密排列,呈不同的断面,细胞和基质成分少,多为成纤维细胞。皮下组织可见大量脂肪细胞聚集形成脂肪小叶,即脂肪组织。其间为疏松结缔组织。脂肪细胞圆形或多边形,空泡状,其胞质和细胞核被挤到边缘,形成淡红色新月形的胞质和扁圆形的胞核。

(3) 观察要点:胶原纤维的排列、脂肪细胞。

三、思考题

1. 在光镜下,致密结缔组织和疏松结缔组织有什么不同?
2. 固有结缔组织有哪几种?
3. 结缔组织的一般特征是什么? 各种纤维和细胞分别有哪些特征?
4. 成纤维细胞和浆细胞的结构和功能有什么不同?
5. 肥大细胞和巨噬细胞的结构和功能有什么不同?

(朱丽娟,李娜)

Chapter 3
Connective Tissue

Ⅰ. Experiment purpose

1. Master the general characteristics and types of connective tissue.

2. Master the features of the collagen fibers, elastic fibers, reticular fiber; fibroblast cells, macrophages, plasma cells, mast cells under the light microscope.

3. Familiar with the structure characteristics and distribution of dense connective tissue, adipose tissue and reticular tissue.

Ⅱ. Experiment contents

1. Loose connective tissue stretched preparation (Fig. 7)

(1) Material and staining: Mesentery (Intraperitoneal injection of trypan blue), HE staining, Neutral Red staining.

(2) Observe:

By eyes: the tissue is stained in light reddish-purple.

Lower power lens: Find an area with light staining. Fibers are thick and thin, criss-crossing and arranges loosely. The pink belt-like fibers are collagen fibers. The purple thin fibers are elastic fibers always with branch. Between the fibers there are a number of cells.

Higher power lens: Focus on two types of cells and the two types of fibers.

① Collagen fibers: In larger quantities, fibers dyed pink are thick and thin, criss-crossing and arranges loosely.

② Elastic fiber: Fiber like fine line, is dyed purple blue and slender, diffraction and branch. The terminal is often curving.

③ Fibroblasts: The largest number of flat-shaped cells. There are more processes. Cells are not very clear outline. Nuclear is larger oval, dyeing shallow, with a clear nucleolus. Cytoplasm is weak basophilic and not clearly.

④ Macrophages: Large, irregular shape. Nuclear small, deep-staining. Cytoplasm is eosinophilic, with varying sizes, uneven distribution of blue particles.

(3) Observation key points: Collagen fiber, elastic fiber, fibroblast and macrophage.

2. Loose connective tissue, dense connective tissue and adipose tissue (Fig. 8)

(1) Material and staining: Palmar skin, HE staining.

(2) Observe:

By eyes: In the superficial indigo blue's part is the epidermis, underneath the epidermis the red part is the dermis, underneath the dermis is the subcutaneous tissue (loose connective tissue and adipose tissue).

Lower power lens: After finding the dermis, observe the dense connective tissue, then move again to the depth portion, observe the loose connective tissue and the fatty tissue.

Higher power lens: In the dermis, within the dense connective tissue a particularly large number of fibers are observed, which are large, with close arranges, and less cells and matrix components.

In subcutaneous tissue, loose connective tissue and adipose tissue can be seen. This part is stained light because of less collagen fiber and elastic fiber. Adipose tissue is mainly gathered from a large number of fat cells, in which there is loose connective tissue.

Larger fat cells are spherical shape, the cytoplasm containing lipid droplets in varying sizes and eventually fused into a big fat droplets located in the central to push the cytoplasm and nuclear to the side.

(3) Observation key points: Collagen fiber, fat cell.

III. Questions

1. What are the differences between the loose connective tissue and dense connective tissue in the general characteristics under the microscope?

2. How many types does the connective tissue have?

3. What is the structural feature of the connective tissue? How to identify several major fibers and cells?

4. What are the features of fibroblasts and plasma cells in the structure and function?

5. What are the features of macrophages and mast cells in the structure and function?

(Zhu Lijuan, Li Na)

第四章
软 骨 和 骨

一、实验目的

1. 掌握透明软骨和长骨的结构特征。
2. 熟悉弹性软骨的结构特征。

二、实验内容

1. 透明软骨 (Hyaline cartilage)(彩图 9～10)

(1) 取材和染色:气管横切面，HE 染色。
(2) 观察:
肉眼:可见紫蓝色"C"形的透明软骨环或软骨片。
低倍:从软骨的表面向内部观察。
① 软骨膜:致密结缔组织,位于软骨表面,HE 染色呈淡红色的。
② 软骨细胞:靠近软骨膜为幼稚软骨细胞,细胞体积较小,扁圆形,单个分布;靠近中央的为成熟软骨细胞,体积渐大,呈圆形或椭圆形,常成群分布,因其由同一幼稚细胞分裂而来,位于同一个软骨陷窝内,故称同源细胞群。
③ 基质:均质状,HE 染色呈成蓝色,软骨陷窝周围染色较深,称软骨囊。软骨内无血管。
高倍:软骨细胞位于骨基质的软骨陷窝中,大多属于同源细胞群。图中上半部分染成淡紫色的是软骨膜。软骨组织中可以观察到不同分化阶段的软骨细胞。在透明软骨的外周,分化早期的软骨细胞呈椭圆形,长轴与软骨表面平行,而在透明软骨的深部,主要是成熟的圆形软骨细胞。
(3) 观察要点: 识别软骨膜、软骨囊、软骨细胞和基质、同源软骨群。

2. 骨组织 (Bone tissue)(彩图 11～12)

(1) 取材和染色:长骨骨干横截面磨片,大丽紫染色。

(2) 观察：

肉眼:为一灰黑色组织。

低倍:

① 骨单位:又称哈弗斯系统,镜下为同心圆排列的板层结构。骨单位中央的圆形空腔为中央管,染色过程中被磨石粉填塞呈黑色,周围围绕以中央管为轴心排列的数层骨板。

② 间骨板:是位于骨单位之间排列不规则的骨板。在骨的内外表面有数层骨板环绕骨干排列,分别称为内、外环骨板。

高倍:仔细调换 40×高倍镜观察,可见骨板之间和骨板上有许多深黑色椭圆形结构,即骨陷窝。由骨陷窝向外发射出的小细管为骨小管。骨陷窝和骨小管是骨细胞的胞体和突起所在部位。相邻骨陷窝的骨小管相互连通。

(3) 观察要点:识别骨单位、间骨板、骨小管、骨陷窝、骨细胞。

三、思考题

1. 试述软骨的组织结构及软骨细胞的光镜结构特点。

2. 试述骨组织中各种细胞的结构和功能。

(吴晓菁,黄少萍)

Chapter 4
Cartilage and Bone

Ⅰ. Experiment purpose

1. Master the classifications and structures of different types of cartilage. Master the structures of the chondrocyte.

2. Master the construction features of the cartilage and the compact bone.

Ⅱ. Experiment contents

1. Hyaline cartilage (Figs. 9-10)

(1) Material: Trachea, HE staining.

(2) Observe:

By eyes: Obviously in the trachea wall can be seen a C-shaped blue hyaline cartilage ring.

Lower power lens:

① Perichondrium: the perichondrium, which belong to dense connective tissue is observed at the surface of the cartilage, and is stained into pink color.

② Chondrocytes: Chondrocytes are located in matrix lacunae, and most belong to isogenous groups. Note the gradual differentiation of cells from the perichondrium into chondrocytes.

③ Matrix: Matrix is homogeneous shape, dyed blue. The matrix dyed deeply around the dimple.

Higher power lens: Chondrocytes are located in matrix lacunae, and most belong to isogenous groups. The upper and lower parts of the figure show the perichondrium stained pink. Note the gradual differentiation of cells from the perichondrium into chondrocytes. At the periphery of hyaline cartilage, young chondrocytes have an elliptic shape, with the long axis parallel to the surface. In the deeper part of the cartilage, cells are more mature and round.

(3) Observation key points: Chondrocytes and isogenous groups of hyaline cartilage, perichondrium.

2. Bone tissue (Figs. 11-12)

(1) Material: Long bone, HE staining.

(2) Observe:

By eyes: the bone tissue is dark grey or black.

Lower power lens: Osteons (Haversian systems) are the basic structural units of compact bone, the Osteons are cylindrical structures between the outer and inner circumferential lamellae.

Higher power lens: They are consisted of a central hole, the Haversian canal, through which blood vessels run and is surrounded by many layers of concentric lamellae. In the lamella, osteocytes can be seen.

(3) Observation key points: identify the osteon, the interstitial lamella, the bone canaliculi, bone lacuna and osteocyte.

III. Questions

1. Describe the structure of the cartilage tissue and the structure of the chondrocyte under the light microscope.

2. Describe the structure and function of four kinds bone cells.

(Wu Xiaojing, Huang Shaoping)

第五章
血　　液

一、实验目的

1. 掌握各种血细胞的光镜形态结构及正常值。
2. 熟悉各种血细胞的电镜结构特征。

二、实验内容

血涂片(Blood smear)(彩图 13～18)

(1) 取材和染色:手指末梢血液,瑞氏染色。

(2) 标本制作:使用75%的乙醇棉球消毒手指,待干后用已消毒的采血器迅速刺入皮肤。第一滴血弃去不用,将第二滴血滴在载玻片上。用盖玻片的一端放在有血液的载玻片上,成45°角,然后推片向右移动,使之与血滴接触,待血滴沿盖玻片的边缘分散后将盖玻片向反方向推动,形成薄薄的血膜。血膜晾干后滴加Wright染液,染色3 min左右,然后滴加等量的磷酸缓冲液,轻轻吹动,使染液与缓冲液充分混合。继续染色5～10 min后,用自来水轻轻冲洗洗,晾干后封片观察。

(3) 观察:

肉眼:玻片上可见粉红色铺成膜状的血组织。

低倍:镜下选择血细胞没有重叠、白细胞较多的部位,转入40×物镜观察。

高倍:按一定方向移动载物台,逐步进行观察。

① 红细胞:数量最多。红细胞染色呈红色,双面凹的圆盘状,无细胞核,中央染色较浅,周围染色较深。

② 中性粒细胞:占白细胞总数的50%～70%,是数量最多的白细胞。细胞呈圆形,细胞核蓝紫色,分2～5叶,叶间以狭窄部相连。胞浆呈粉红色,内含许多细小而均匀的淡紫红色颗粒。

③ 淋巴细胞:占白细胞总数的20%～30%。细胞呈圆形,大小不一。细胞核为椭圆形或圆形,蓝紫色,胞浆很少,仅在细胞核周围形成窄带,有少量淡粉色嗜天青颗粒。

④ 嗜酸性粒细胞：占白细胞总数的0.5%～3%。细胞呈圆形，细胞核为蓝紫色，常分成两叶，叶间有狭窄部相连。胞浆染成粉红色，胞浆中充满粗大而均匀的嗜酸性颗粒。

⑤ 嗜碱性粒细胞：占白细胞总数的0～1%。细胞呈圆形，细胞核多为"S"形或不规则形状，着色浅。胞浆中含大量嗜碱性颗粒，呈深蓝紫色，将细胞核遮盖，因此细胞核轮廓不清晰。

⑥ 单核细胞：占白细胞总数的3%～8%；细胞体积较大，细胞核多为马蹄形或者肾形，细胞核常偏在细胞一边，胞浆常染成浅灰蓝色。

⑦ 血小板：聚集成群，为骨髓巨核细胞上脱落下来的胞浆小块，胞质中有紫红色颗粒，胞质周边部的染色为浅蓝色。大量血小板聚集时，血小板的轮廓会不清晰。

(4) 观察要点：识别红细胞以及各种白细胞。

三、思考题

1. 白细胞的分类原则是什么？各类白细胞的正常值和百分比是多少？
2. 试述各类白细胞的光镜结构特点和功能。
3. 光镜下如何区分中性粒细胞和嗜酸性粒细胞？如何区分淋巴细胞和单核细胞？

(吴晓菁，黄少萍)

Chapter 5
Blood

Ⅰ. Experiment purpose

1. Master the normal number and percentage of each type of white blood cell.

2. Master the light microscope morphology and the function of each type of white blood cell.

3. Master the electron microscopic structure of each of white blood cell.

Ⅱ. Experiment contents

Blood smear (Figs. 13-18)

(1) Material: Person's blood, Wright's staining;

(2) preparation of the Blood smear: Clean the finger with 75% ethyl alcohol. Use the sterilized hemostix to take the blood. Abandon the first drop. Clean glass slide on a flat surface. Add one small drop of blood to one end. Take another clean slide, and holding at an angle of about 45 degree, touch the blood with one end of the slide so the blood runs along the edge of the slide by capillary action. Push carefully along the length of the first slide to produce a thin smear of blood. Dry out the blood smear and add Wight liquor to stain for 3 min, add phosphate buffer to mix the Wight liquor together and stain for 5-10 min. Wash by water carefully and cover the slide.

(3) Observe:

By eyes: Choose the site of the blood thinner film

Lower power lens: Choice the parts in without overlapping, evenly distributed blood cells and more interleukin.

Higher power lens:

Moving slice according to a certain direction and observing step-by-step.

① Erythrocytes (red blood cells): In larger quantities, the cells of the Erythrocytesare biconcave disks without nuclei. The cells are dyed orange, the central color light, around the color depth, diameter about 7 μm.

② Neutrophils: Neutrophils constitute 60%-70% of circulating leukocytes. They are 10-12 μm in diameter (in blood smears), with a nucleus consisting of 2-5(usually 3) lobes linked by fine threads of chromatin. Cytoplasm is pink, which contain many small, lavender uniform particles.

③ Eosinophils: Eosinophils constitute 0.5%-3% of circulating leukocytes. In the blood smears, Eosinophils are about the same size as neutrophil and contain a classic bilobed nucleus. The main characteristic of the Eosinophils is the presence of many large and evenly distributed refractile specific granules that are stained by eosin.

④ Basophils: Basophils make up less than 1% of blood leukocytes and are therefore difficult to find in smears of normal blood. They are about 10-11 μm in diameter. Specific granules in basophils are fewer and more irregular in size and shape than the granules of the other granulocytes. Cells are round. The nucleus of the Basophils are S-shaped or irregular-shaped. Since the cytoplasm is filed with specific granules, the nucleus of the Basophils are usually obscure.

⑤ Lymphocytes: Lymphocytes have difference size. Lymphocytes with diameters of 6-8 μm are known as small lymphocytes. The small lymphocyte, which is predominant in the blood, has a spherical nucleus, sometimes with an indentation. Its chromatin is condensed and appears as coarse clumps, as a result the nucleus is intensely stained in the usual preparations and facilitates the identification of the lymphocyte. The cytoplasm of the small lymphocyte is scanty, in blood smears it appears as a thin rim around the nucleus.

⑥ Monocytes: Monocytes constitute 0.5%-3% of circulating leukocytes with diameters varying from 14-20 μm. The nucleus are oval, horseshoe-, or kidney-shaped and are generally eccentrically placed. The nuclei of monocytes stain lighter than that of large lymphocytes. The cytoplasm of the monocyte is basophilic and frequently contains very fine azurophilic granules (lysosomes), some of which are at the limit of the light microscope's resolution. These granules are distributed through the cytoplasm, giving it a bluish-gray color in stained smears.

⑦ Platelet: gather in groups, for marrow megakaryocyte falls off cytoplasmic small piece, there are purplish red granule in cytoplasm, cytoplasm circumferential ministry stain is shallow blue. When large Numbers of platelets accumulate, the outline of the platelets is not clear.

(4) Observation key points: Identify the structures of red blood cells and various types of white blood cells.

III. Questions

1. What is the classification principle of leucocyte? What is the normal number and percentage of different kinds of leukocyte?

2. Describe the structure and function of various types of the leukocytes.

3. How to distinguish the structures of eosinophils and neutrophils under light microscope? How to distinguish the structures of lymphocytes and monocytes under light microscope?

(Wu Xiaojing, Huang Shaoping)

第六章
肌 肉 组 织

一、实验目的

1. 掌握骨骼肌、心肌和平滑肌在纵、横切面的形态结构特点。
2. 能够识别闰盘。

二、实验内容

1. 骨骼肌(Skeleton muscle)(彩图 19～20)

(1) 取材和染色:骨骼肌,HE 染色。
(2) 观察:
肉眼:可见红色的骨骼肌组织。
低倍:① 纵切面的骨骼肌肌纤维呈长纤维状,平行排列,肌纤维之间有少量结缔组织,为肌内膜。骨骼肌细胞的边缘能观察到每个细胞都有多个细胞核。
② 横切面上骨骼肌肌细胞呈圆形或者多边形,每一个肌细胞周围都有少量的肌内膜包裹。
高倍:① 骨骼肌纵切面上:明暗交替排列的周期性横纹,即明带和暗带。
② 骨骼肌横切面:能观察到圆点状的肌原纤维。细胞核多位于细纤维边缘贴近肌内膜的区域,呈红色点状。
(3) 观察要点:在纵切面上观察横纹、细胞形态和细胞核数量及位置,横切面上观察细胞形态及肌原纤维断面。

2. 心肌 (Cardiac muscle)(彩图 21～22)

(1) 取材和染色:心脏, HE 染色。
(2) 观察:
肉眼:肉眼下,心肌为一片染色较红的组织块
低倍:① 纵切面呈短杆状,有分支相,大多数心肌细胞只有 1 个细胞核,少数有 2 个

细胞核，位于心肌的中央。

② 横切面为大小不等的团块。细胞之间有少量结缔组织。

高倍：①纵切面上可见横纹，但不如骨骼肌明显。

② 相邻心肌细胞之间有闰盘，为一条颜色较深的、与横纹平行的细线。心肌细胞核周围由于肌丝较少，故染色淡。胞质内的横纹不如骨髓肌清晰。横切面为形态不规则的团块，核位于中央。

（3）观察要点：在纵切面上观察横纹、心肌细胞的分支以及闰盘，纵切面上观察肌原纤维。观察纵、横切面的结构差异。

3. 平滑肌（Smooth muscle）（彩图 23～24）

（1）取材和染色：消化管，HE 染色。

（2）观察：

肉眼：位于消化管壁靠近外层的区域，呈淡红色。

低倍：找到染色较红的肌层，在片中可清楚见到平滑肌的纵切、横切断面。

高倍：平滑肌纵切面：细胞呈长梭形，两端尖细，中部较粗，细胞核短杆状，居中，胞质嗜酸性。平滑机横切面：可见大小不一的圆形结构。大的横断面上能够观察到居中的细胞核，小的切面上没有细胞核。

（3）观察要点：观察平滑肌的纵、横切面，观察细胞核。

三、思考题

1. 试述骨骼肌的电镜结构特点。

2. 试述骨骼肌、心肌、平滑肌在光镜下的纵、横切面结构特点。

（吴晓菁，黄少萍）

Chapter 6
Muscle Tissue

Ⅰ. Experiment purpose

1. Master the morphology of longitudinal section and transverse section of skeletal muscle, cardiac muscle and smooth muscle.

2. Familiar with the structure characteristics and distribution of cardiac muscle intercalated disk.

Ⅱ. Experiment contents

1. Skeletal muscle (Figs. 19-20)

(1) Material: Tongue, HE staining;

(2) Observe:

By eyes: The tissue is dyed red.

Lower power lens:

① Cells are long cylindrical in longitudinal section and parallel arrangement, the connective tissue is observed between muscle fibers and named as endomysium Most of the skeletal muscle cell has multiple nuclei.

② Cells are round or polygon in transvers section. connective tissue is observed surrounding the muscle fiber.

Higher power lens:

① Longitudinal section: Skeletal muscle consists of muscle fibers, bundles of very long (up to 30 cm) cylindrical multinucleated cells with a diameter of 10-100 μm.The oval nuclei are usually found at the periphery of the cell under the cell membrane. The muscle fiber shows cross-striations of alternating light and dark bands.

② Transverse section: Cell are round, basically the same size, The oval nuclei are at the periphery of the cell under the cell membrane. Myofibrils are red punctate.

2. Cardiac muscle (Figs. 21-22)

(1) Material: Heart, HE staining.

(2) Observe:

By eyes: A dyed red tissue.

Lower power lens: Cells are short cylindrical in longitudinal section and may branch at their ends to form connections with adjacent cells. Cell are mass that size does not equal in transverse section.

Higher power lens:

Longitudinal section: Cells are short cylindrical and exhibit a cross—striated banding pattern identical to that of skeletal muscle, but not very clear. Each cardiac muscle cell possesses only one or two centrally located pale-staining nuclei. On cardiac muscle there are the presence of dark-staining transverse lines known as the intercalated disc that cross the chains of cardiac cells at irregular intervals. The junctions may appear as straight lines or may exhibit a steplike pattern.

Transverse section: Cell are mass that size is not equal and shape is irregular in transverse section.

(3) Observation key points: striation, the branch of the myocardium and intercalated disc in longitudinal sections.

3. Smooth muscle (Figs. 23-24)

(1) Material: Digestive tract, HE staining.

(2) Observe:

By eyes: A dyed red tissue in the wall of digestive tract.

Lower power lens: Finding some parts of red dye, the longitudinal section and transverse section of smooth muscle will be seen clear.

Higher power lens:

Longitudinal section: Cells are long fusiform and largest at their midpoints and taper toward their ends. Each cell has a single nucleus located in the center of the broadest part of the cell. Cytoplasm is eosinophilic

Transverse section: Since the different parts of the muscle cells cut, so we can see large and small circular structure. Nucleus can be seen in large circular structure that nucleus cut in the central.

(3) Observation key points: find the nuclei in longitudinal and transvers sections.

Ⅲ. Questions

1. Describe the structural characters of skeletal muscle by electron microscopy.

2. Describe the structural characters of skeletal musclel, cardiac muscle, smooth muscle in longitudinal and transverse section under the light microscope.

(Wu Xiaojing, Huang Shaoping)

第七章
神 经 组 织

一、实验目的

1. 掌握神经元的光镜结构特点。

2. 掌握有髓神经纤维的纵、横切面结构特点。

二、实验内容

1. 多极神经元（Multipolar neuron)(彩图 25～26)

(1) 取材和染色:脊髓,HE 染色。

(2) 观察

肉眼:脊髓横切面上,有中央管和灰质,其中灰质呈蝴蝶状,灰质周围的浅染部分为白质。灰质腹侧较粗短的部分为前角。

低倍:脊髓前角内可见胞体大小不一、突起较多的多边形细胞,核大,染色深。

高倍:细胞核位于神经元中央,染色深,核膜和核仁均清晰可见。胞体向四周伸出许多突起,为树突和轴突。神经元可有一个或多个树突,其中有尼氏体,但是轴突只有一根且没有尼氏体。轴突的起始部称为轴丘,呈锥圆形,染色浅。

(3) 观察要点:观察神经元的胞体、细胞核、尼氏小体、树突和轴突。区分树突和轴突。

2. 有髓神经纤维(Myelinated nerve fibers)(彩图 27～30)

(1) 取材和染色:坐骨神经, HE 染色。

(2) 观察:

肉眼:神经纤维纵切面为长条状结构,神经纤维横切面为圆形。

低倍:① 纵切面上可见平行排列的红色条纹,即有髓神经纤维。神经外有结缔组织包裹,称为神经外膜。

② 横切面上神经最外周能观察到一圈结缔组织,即为神经外膜;内侧有成束分布的

神经。

高倍:① 纵切面上轴突位于有髓神经纤维中部,为一条紫色的粗线,髓鞘包裹在轴突外周,染色较浅。由于制片时髓鞘的脂质溶解,因此呈网状空泡状;髓鞘中断处会形成狭窄的郎飞结,相邻的两个郎飞结之间的轴膜暴露在外,称为结间体。

② 横切面上神经的最外层是神经外膜,染色为红色,神经外膜内有成束分布的神经纤维,束外包裹的结缔组织为神经束膜;单个神经纤维则为神经束中的小圆圈,圆圈中心的蓝色或灰色的圆点即为轴突横切面。施万细胞包裹在轴突外,边缘染色红色,为髓鞘的蛋白结构。此外在髓鞘和轴突之间能够观察到红色细网状蛋白质。

(3) 观察要点:在纵切面上观察轴突和郎飞结。在横切面上观察轴突、髓鞘、神经外膜、神经束膜等结构。

三、思考题

1. 试述多极神经元的光镜结构特点。
2. 描述有髓神经纤维横切面和纵切面的形态结构。

(夏江燕,黄少萍)

Chapter 7
Nerve Tissue

Ⅰ. Experiment purpose

(1) Master the construction features of neurons.

(2) Master the structural charactens of the myelinated nerve fibers in transverse and longitudinal section.

Ⅱ. Experiment contents

1. Multipolar Neuron (Figs. 25-26)

(1) Material: spinal cord, HE staining.

(2) Observe:

By eyes: In the transverse section of spinal cord, gray matter deeper stained is shaped like a butterfly in the central.

Lower power lens: In slender processes of gray matter the neurons known as motor neurons are large cell body, more cell processes and purple cytoplasm.

Higher power lens: Most nerve cells have a spherical, large, euchromatic (pale staining) nucleus with a prominent nucleolus. In the dendrites and cell body, the basophilic granular areas called Nissl bodies. Nissl bodies only exist in the dendritic and cell body. Many processes extend to the surrounding from cell body that are the dendrites and only one axon.

(3) Observation key points: Observe the cell body, nuclei, Nissl body, axons and dendrites of the neuron. Differentiate the axon from the dendrite.

2. Myelinated nerve fibers (Figs. 27-30)

(1) Materials: Sciatic nerve, HE staining.

(2) Observe:

By eyes: The long fiber is the longitudinal section of the nerve fiber, the round one is the transverse section of the nerve fiber.

Lower power lens:

① Longitudinal section: Many long strip-like myelinated fibers is red. The whole nerve fiber is surrounded by the connective tissue, called epineurium.

② Transverse section: Nerve is surrounded by the epineurium, in the interior, there are several bundles of nerve fibers, is surrounded by the perineurium. A single nerve fiber inside the perineurium is surrounded by the endoneurium.

Higher power lens:

① Longitudinal section: In the center of the fiber, is the axon, in purple. The myelin sheath surround the axon, and outside the sheath is the neurilemma, like a thin red line. Inside the neurilemma there are some Schwann cells' ovoid nuclei. The myelin sheath is interrupted by the gap called the nodes of Ranvier. The distance between two Ranvier called the internode.

② Transverse section: The outer line of transverse section of myelinated fiber like red circle line, called epineurium. As shown in a purple spot, the axon is observed in the center of the fiber. The myelin sheath is located between the epineurium and the axon.

(3) Observation key points: Observe the node of Ranvier and axon in longitudinal section. Observe the axon and myelin sheath, epineurium, perineurium and endoneurium in transverse section.

Ⅲ. Questions

1. Describe the structure of the multipolar neuron under the light microscope.

2. Describe the longitudinal and transverse section of the myelinated nerve fiber respectively.

(Xia Jiangyan, Huang Shaoping)

第八章
循 环 系 统

一、实验目的

1. 掌握中动脉、大动脉管壁的结构特点。

2. 掌握心脏壁的三层结构，浦肯野纤维的结构特点，区分心内膜和心外膜。

3. 熟悉静脉的结构特点。

二、实验内容

1. 中动脉（Medium artery）（彩图 31～32）

（1）取材和染色：中动脉和中静脉，HE 染色。

（2）观察：

肉眼：可见 2 个管腔横切面，中动脉腔小而圆，管壁厚；中静脉腔大而不规则，管壁薄。

低倍：找到中动脉，三层结构清晰可辨。① 靠近管腔可见一波浪状、折光性强的亮粉红色条带，为内弹性膜（internal elastic lamina），近腔面部分为内膜。② 向外可见粉红色的肌性中膜。③ 最外层为浅染的结缔组织外膜，厚度与中膜近似，中膜和外膜之间可见不连续的外弹性膜（external elastic lamina）。④ 找到伴行的中静脉，与中动脉相比较，其管壁薄，内外弹性膜不明显或阙如，三层结构分界不明显，中膜薄，结缔组织外膜厚。

高倍：由内向外依次详细观察中动脉的三层结构。

① 内膜：ⅰ 内皮：为单层扁平上皮。ⅱ 内皮下层：为一层薄而细密的结缔组织。ⅲ 内弹性膜：清晰可辨，为一条波浪状的亮粉红色条带。

② 中膜：较厚，约占整个管壁厚度的一半，为 10～40 层环形平滑肌纤维构成。

③ 外膜：厚度和中膜大致相等，为疏松结缔组织，可见外弹性膜，为不连续的波浪状亮粉红色条带，不如内弹性膜发达；在外膜中还可见脂肪细胞和营养血管（小动脉和小静脉）。

（3）观察要点：区分三层结构，辨认内膜各层，内弹性膜、外弹性膜、肌性中膜等。

2. 大动脉（Large artery）（彩图 33～34）

（1）取材和染色：大动脉，HE 染色。

(2) 观察:

肉眼:可见内膜、外膜较薄,浅粉红色;中膜较厚,染色深。

低倍:与中动脉比较,内膜较中动脉厚,为浅粉红色;中膜最厚,为多层波浪状的亮粉红色条带,为弹性蛋白构成的弹性膜;外膜薄,为浅粉红色的较致密结缔组织,内、外弹性膜不明显。

高倍:由内向外依次详细观察。

① 内膜:内皮下层较中动脉厚,内弹性膜与中膜的弹性膜相接,故不易分辨。

② 中膜:最厚,可见40~70层亮粉红色的波浪状弹性膜,之间含少量胶原纤维、弹性纤维和少量平滑肌。

③ 外膜:较薄;为较致密结缔组织,无明显外弹性膜。

(3) 观察要点:区分三层结构,辨认内膜各层,内弹性膜、中膜和外弹性膜。

3. 心脏 (Heart)(彩图35~36)

(1) 取材和染色:心脏,HE染色。

(2) 观察:

肉眼:可见较厚的心脏壁,中间的心肌膜最厚,染色为深红色,两侧为较薄的心内膜与心外膜,染色为浅粉红色。

低倍:首先鉴别心内膜与心外膜,两者均为浅染的结缔组织,位于心肌膜的两侧。在心外膜中可以看到脂肪组织和血管,则心肌膜的另一侧为心内膜,心内膜靠近心肌膜处可见大而浅染的束细胞(浦肯野纤维,Purkinje fiber)。然后观察心肌膜,辨别心肌纤维的横、纵和斜断面。

高倍:由内向外依次详细观察。

① 心内膜:ⅰ内皮:与血管的内皮相延续;ⅱ内皮下层:薄层结缔组织,含少量平滑肌;ⅲ心内膜下层:疏松结缔组织,可见束细胞,比普通心肌纤维短而粗,胞质染色淡,1~2个细胞核在中央。

② 心肌膜:最厚,由三层心肌纤维构成,辨别其横、纵和斜断面;肌束间为结缔组织和丰富的毛细血管。

③ 心外膜:由疏松结缔组织和外层的间皮构成,结缔组织中可见脂肪细胞、小动脉和小静脉。

(3) 观察要点:区分三层结构,区分心内膜和心外膜,辨认浦肯野纤维。

三、思考题

1. 中动脉和大动脉的结构特点是什么?大动脉和中动脉最主要的区别在哪?
2. 光镜下如何区分心脏壁的心内膜和心外膜?

(陆静,黄少萍)

Chapter 8
Circulatory System

Ⅰ. Experiment purpose

1. To master the structure of the wall in medium arteries and large arteries.

2. To master the structure of the wall in heart and the key features of the Purkinje fibers. Differentiate the endocardium from the epicardium.

3. To have an intimate knowledge of the structure of the veins.

Ⅱ. Experiment contents

1. Medium artery (Figs. 31-32)

(1) Material and staining: Medium artery and medium vein, HE staining.

(2) Observe:

By eyes: Two lumen structures can be seen. The lumen of the artery is smaller and round and its wall is thicker. The vein's lumen is larger and irregular and its wall is thinner.

Lower power lens: The three layers of the medium artery can be distinguished clearly. ① The internal elastic lamina is stained red and waved-shape, it is the marker between the tunic intima and tunic media. ② The tunic media is composed of smooth muscle cells. ③ The tunic adventitia is composed of connective tissue and stained pink. The thickness of the tunic media and tunic adventitia are almost the same. Between the tunic media and tunic adventitia, we can see discontinuous external elastic lamina. ④ Compared with artery, the wall of the accompanying vein is thinner, internal and external elastic lamina are indistinct, and three layers cannot be distinguished clearly.

Higher power lens: Observe the three layers of the medium artery carefully.

① Tunic intima: ⅰ Endothelium: a simple squamous epithelium bordering the lumen. ⅱ Subendothelial layer: composed of a thin layer of connective tissue.

ⅲ Internal elastic lamina: stained red, waved-shape.

② Tunic media: thick, consists mainly of circumferential vascular smooth muscle fibers, about 10-40 layers.

③ Tunic adventitia: composed of loose connective tissue, discontinuous, red, waved-shaped external elastic lamina lies between the media and the tunica adventitia, fat cells and vasa vasorum (small blood vessels) can be seen.

(3) Observation key points: Distinguish the three layers, internal elastic lamina, external elastic lamina, the muscular membrane.

2. Large artery (Figs. 33-34)

(1) Material and staining: Large artery, HE staining.

(2) Observe:

By eyes: The tunic intima and tunic adventitia are stained pink and thinner, the tunic media is stained dark pink and thicker.

Lower power lens: Compared with the medium artery, the tunic intima is thicker and stained pink, the tunic media is composed of many layers of concentric, fenestrated elastic laminae, the tunic adventitia is composed of connective tissue and stained pink. Compared with the medium artery, the internal and external elastic lamina cannot be distinguished clearly.

Higher power lens: Observe the three layers of the large artery carefully.

① Tunic intima: The subendothelial layer is thicker than that of the medium artery, the internal elastic lamina is adjacent to the elastic lamina of the tunic media, so it is hard to be distinguished clearly.

② Tunic media: Thick, contains 40 - 70 layers of red, waved elastic laminae, alternating with circularly oriented smooth muscle cells, collagen fibers and elastic fibers.

③ Tunic adventitia: Contains a thin layer of connective tissue, external elastic lamina is not obvious.

(3) Observation key points: Distinguish the three layers, internal elastic lamina external elastic lamina, the muscular membrane.

3. Heart (Figs. 35-36)

(1) Material and staining: Heart, HE staining.

(2) Observe:

By eyes: The wall of the heart is thick. The myocardium is the thickest middle layer and stained dark pink, flanking are thinner endocardium and epicardium and stained light pink.

Lower power lens: First discriminate the endocardium from the epicardium, they are both connective tissue and covered by a single layer of squamous endothelial cells. There are Purkinje cells in the endocardium, yet the epicardium contains some fat cells and vessels. In the myocardium, cardiac muscle cells are arranged in three directions.

Higher power lens:

① Endocardium: ⅰ endothelium. ⅱ subendothial layer: a thin layer of connective tissue, contains several smooth muscle cells. ⅲ subendocardial layer: loose connective tissue, contains Purkinje cells, which are larger and shorter than normal cardiac muscle cells and stained pale. The nuclear is small and cytoplasm is rich.

② Myocardium: the thickest layer, cardiac muscle cells are arranged in three directions. Connective tissue and capillaries can be seen among cardiac muscle fibers.

③ Epicardium: loose connective tissue, contains some fat cells and vessels, such as small arteries and small veins. The epicardium is covered by a single layer of epithelium cells.

(3) Observation key points: Distinguish the three layers, endocardium, epicardium, Purkinje fibers.

III. Questions

1. What are the general characters of the organs of arteries? What is the main difference among larger artery and medium artery?

2. How to distinguish the endocardium and the epicardium under the light microscopy?

(Lu Jing, Huang Shaoping)

第九章
免 疫 系 统

一、实验目的

1. 掌握淋巴结、脾和胸腺的组织结构。
2. 掌握淋巴小结的结构特点。
3. 掌握弥散淋巴组织的结构特点。

二、实验内容

1. 淋巴结（Lymph node）（彩图 37～38）

（1）取材和染色：淋巴结，HE 染色。

（2）观察：

肉眼：可见 1 个染成紫红色的椭圆形组织，周边染色深，为淋巴结的皮质（cortex），中央染色浅，为髓质（medulla）。

低倍：淋巴结表面为结缔组织构成的被膜（capsule），被膜结缔组织深入淋巴结实质形成小梁（trabecular），切片上为多个粉红色的不规则断面。实质分为外周深染的皮质和中央浅染的髓质。

① 皮质：分为浅层皮质、副皮质区和皮质淋巴窦（lymphatic sinuses）。被膜下方为浅层皮质，主要由淋巴小结（lymphoid nodules）构成，初级淋巴小结为椭圆形结构，被染成均一的蓝紫色，主要由 B 淋巴细胞构成；有的淋巴小结中央染色浅，称为生发中心（germinal center），这样的淋巴小结又叫作次级淋巴小结。浅层皮质的下方为副皮质区，为弥散淋巴组织，主要由 T 淋巴细胞构成。皮质淋巴窦又分为被膜下方的被膜下淋巴窦（subcapsular sinus）和小梁周围的小梁周窦（peritrabecular sinus）。

② 髓质：位于淋巴结中央，皮质的深部，由髓索（medullary cord）和髓窦（medullary sinus）构成，髓索染色深，为淋巴组织构成的条索状结构，并相互连接成网，髓索之间浅染的区域为髓窦，与皮质淋巴窦相通。

高倍：

① 淋巴小结：主要由淋巴细胞构成，还有少量的巨噬细胞和网状细胞。淋巴细胞体

积小，染成蓝紫色；巨噬细胞体积较大，胞质染成红色；网状细胞分界不清，呈星形，胞质染成淡粉红色，胞核体积大，染色浅。

② 髓索：由密集的淋巴细胞、散在的巨噬细胞、网状细胞构成。

③ 淋巴窦：窦壁由内皮覆盖，窦腔内可见散在的网状细胞、淋巴细胞和巨噬细胞，细胞分界清楚，较易辨认。

(3) 观察要点：区分淋巴结各部；观察淋巴小结、髓索；观察淋巴窦的结构及巨噬细胞等。

2. 脾（Spleen）（彩图 39～40）

(1) 取材和染色：脾，HE 染色。

(2) 观察：

肉眼：可见深红色三角形组织，为脾的切面，组织中散在染成蓝色的小点，为白髓（white pulp），其他红色组织为红髓（red pulp）。

低倍：被膜较厚，染成粉红色，由间皮和结缔组织构成，表面光滑，结缔组织中含有平滑肌纤维。被膜深入实质形成脾小梁，有分支，散在分布于实质内，内含小梁动脉、小梁静脉。实质中可见散在的染成蓝紫色的白髓，其他部分为染成红色的红髓。

① 白髓：散在分布于实质内，为紫蓝色椭圆形结构，由脾小结（splenic corpuscle）、中央动脉（central artery）和动脉周围淋巴鞘（periarterial lymphatic sheaths）构成。脾小结与淋巴小结结构类似，脾小结边缘可见血管断面，为中央动脉，中央动脉周围的弥散淋巴组织，称为动脉周围淋巴鞘。脾小结主要由 B 淋巴细胞构成。动脉周围淋巴鞘主要由 T 淋巴细胞构成。

② 红髓：实质内除白髓外的其他组织，含有丰富的血细胞，故呈红色，由脾索（splenic cords）和脾血窦（splenic sinusoids）构成。脾索为条索状分支的淋巴组织，主要含 B 淋巴细胞、血细胞和巨噬细胞；脾窦为血窦，充满血细胞，窦壁由长杆状内皮细胞围成，间隙大，基膜不完整。

高倍：重点观察脾血窦的杆状内皮细胞。切片中杆状内皮细胞常呈横断面，窦壁不连续，内皮细胞胞核向窦腔突起。

(3) 观察要点：区分脾脏各部；观察脾小结、中央动脉、脾血窦结构及巨噬细胞等。

3. 胸腺（Thymus）（彩图 41～42）

(1) 取材和染色：胸腺，HE 染色。

(2) 观察：

肉眼：可见蓝紫色的叶状组织，为胸腺。

低倍：外层为结缔组织被膜，被膜深入实质形成小叶间隔（septa），又称为胸腺隔，将实质分成许多不完整的胸腺小叶，每个胸腺小叶外周染色深，为皮质（cortex），中央染色浅，为髓质（medulla），各小叶髓质相连通。髓质中可见粉红色的结构，一般为胸腺小体（Hassall's corpuscle）或血管，需在高倍镜下分辨。

高倍：

① 皮质：以胸腺上皮细胞（上皮性网状细胞）为支架，网眼中有密集的胸腺细胞（T淋巴细胞）、少量巨噬细胞，细胞分界不清。胸腺上皮细胞胞质染色浅粉红色，胞核较大，椭圆形，染色浅。

② 髓质：较多胸腺上皮细胞，少量胸腺细胞和巨噬细胞，细胞分界较皮质清楚；髓质中央可见胸腺小体，由胸腺上皮细胞呈同心圆状排列而成，外层细胞可见细胞核，中层和内层细胞角化，核消失，呈均质状粉红色，注意与髓质中血管区别。

（3）观察要点：区分胸腺各部；辨认上皮性网状细胞、胸腺细胞、胸腺小体等。

三、思考题

1. 淋巴结的结构特征是什么？

2. 淋巴窦的结构和功能是什么？脾窦的结构和功能是什么？

3. 光镜下如何区别淋巴结、脾和胸腺？

（张昕昕，黄少萍）

Chapter 9
Immune System

Ⅰ. Experiment purpose

1. To master the histological structure of the lymph node, spleen and thymus.
2. To master the key structures of lymphatic nodules.
3. To master the key structures of diffuse lymphatic tissues.

Ⅱ. Experiment contents

1. Lymph node (Figs. 37-38)

(1) Material and staining: Lymphoid node, HE staining.

(2) Observe:

By eyes: A purple-stained ovoid tissue can be seen, the peripheral dark zone is known as the cortex, and the central part as medulla.

Lower power lens: Connective tissue membrane covers the surface of the lymph node, and send trabeculae into its parenchyma. Sections in different directions of the trabeculae can be seen. The parenchyma of the lymph node is divided into the outer cortex and inner medulla.

① Cortex: It consists of three zones: the peripheral cortex, the paracortical zone and the lymphatic sinuses. The peripheral cortex is under the capsule, and mainly consist lymphoid nodules, which are composed of B cells. Primary lymphatic nodules are elliptoid areas of homogeneous density and stained dark blue. Some lymphatic nodules have a paler-staining central area called the germinal center, these are secondary lymphoid nodules. The paracortical zone is composed of diffuse lymphatic tissue and rich in T lymphocytes. Lymphatic sinuses are located under the capsule (subcapsular sinus) and along the trabeculae (peritrabecular sinus).

② Medulla: It is the inner part of the lymph node, consists of medullary cords and medullary sinuses. The medullary cords are stained dark blue and are branched extension the medulla. The medullary cords are separated by the medullary sinuses, which connect with the lymphatic sinuses.

Higher power lens:

① Lymphoid nodules: They are mainly composed of lymphocyte, some macrophages and reticular cells. The lymphocytes are round, small and stained dark blue; the macrophages are large, and the cytoplasm is stained pink; the cytoplasm of the reticular cells are stained light pink, the nuclear are large stained pale; the cells are stellate and the borders are not clear.

② Medullary cords: They are mainly composed of the lymphocytes, macrophages, reticular cells.

③ Lymphatic sinuses: Lymphatic sinuses are lined by endothelial cells, in the sinuses there are reticular cells, lymphocytes and macrophages.

(3) Observation key points: Distinguish every parts of the lymph node, lymphatic nodules, medullary cords, medullary nodules, the cell borders are clear.

2. Spleen (Figs. 39-40)

(1) Material and staining: Spleen, HE staining.

(2) Observe:

By eyes: The tissue is stained dark red, blue spots call white pulp scattered in the tissue, others call red pulp are stained red.

Lower power lens: The spleen is surrounded by a thick pink capsule of mesothelium and dense connective tissue, a few smooth muscle cells can be seen in the connective tissue. From the capsule, trabeculae of connective tissue extend into the parenchyma, arteries and veins can be seen in the trabeculae. White pulps are stained blue and red pulps are stained red.

① White pulps: The white pulps are oval blue white pulps scattered in the parenchyma, consist of splenic corpuscle, central artery and periarterial lymphatic sheaths. The structure of splenic corpuscle is similar to lymphoid nodules, central artery situates on the periphery of splenic corpuscle, the central artery is surrounded by diffuse lymphatic tissue called periarterial lymphatic sheaths. The splenic corpuscle is mainly composed of B cells and the periarterial lymphatic sheaths is mainly composed of T cells.

② Red pulps: The red pulp is tissue between the white pulp and trabecular, it is rich in blood cells and stained red, and has two major components: the splenic cords and the splenic sinusoids. The splenic cords are irregular reticular connective tissue sheets that branch and anastomose to surround the sinuses, mainly consist B cells, blood cells and macrophage. The splenic sinusoids are blood sinuses and filled with blood cells, the wall is covered by rod-shaped endothelial cells, there are spaces between the lining endothelial cells and the basal lamina is discontinuous.

Higher power lens: Observe the rod-shaped endothelial cells carefully. They are mostly presented as transverse section, the wall is discontinuous, and the nuclei of the endothelial cells bulge into the lumen.

(3) Observation key points: Distinguish three parts of the spleen, splenic corpuscle, central artery, splenic sinusoid, macrophage.

3. Thymus (Figs. 41-42)

(1) Material and staining: Thymus, HE staining.

(2) Observe:

By eyes: The blue lobe is the thymus.

Lower power lens: The thymus is covered by a thin connective tissue capsule that penetrates the lobes as septa, dividing the lobe into incomplete lobules. Each lobule has a peripheral dark-staining cortex and a central light-staining medulla. Each lobule's medulla is continuous with that of adjacent lobules. A pink-staining structure can be seen in the medulla, it may be Hassall's corpuscle or blood vessel, can be confirmed at higher power lens.

Higher power lens:

① Cortex: Epithelial reticular cells link to each other, forming a network throughout the cortex, the interspaces of this network are filled with thymic cells and some macrophage, the cell borders are not clear. The epithelial reticular cell has a larger ovoid nuclear in light staining.

② Medulla: Many epithelial reticular cells, some thymic cells and macrophages can be seen, the cell borders are clear. In the center, Hassall's corpuscles can be seen, they are composed of the epithelial reticular cells, and arrange in concentric circles, nucleus can be seen in cell at the out layer while degenerate at the inner layer, which present as homogeneous pink. Distinguish the Hassall's corpuscles from the blood vessels.

(3) Observation key points: epithelial reticular cells, thymic cells, Hassall's corpuscle.

III. Questions

1. What are the key characters of the lymphatic nodules?

2. What is the structure and function of lymphatic sinuses? What is the structure and function of the splenic sinusoids?

3. How to distinguish the lymph node, the spleen and the thymus under the light microscopy?

(Zhang Xinxin, Huang Shaoping)

第十章
皮 肤

一、实验目的

1. 掌握表皮和真皮的分层与结构特点。

2. 熟悉毛、皮脂腺和汗腺的结构特点。

二、实验内容

1. 掌皮（Skin：palm）（彩图 43～46）

（1）取材和染色：掌皮，HE 染色。

（2）观察：

肉眼：可见染成紫色的一层为表皮（epidermis），染成粉红色的为真皮（dermis）和皮下组织部分。

低倍：染成深紫色的一层为表皮，下方染成粉红色的组织为真皮和皮下组织。

① 表皮：为角化的复层扁平上皮，掌皮为厚皮肤，光镜下分为 5 层结构，由深部到表层分别为基底层（stratum basale）、棘层（stratum spinosum）、颗粒层（stratum granulosum）、透明层（stratum lucidum）和角质层（stratum corneum）。ⅰ 基底层：为一层矮柱状或立方形细胞，胞质较少，嗜碱性，胞核卵圆形，染色较深。ⅱ 棘层：由 4～10 层多边形细胞构成，细胞体积大，胞质嗜碱性，胞核大。ⅲ 颗粒层：由 3～5 层梭形细胞构成，胞核趋近退化，胞质内有很多深蓝色颗粒。ⅳ 透明层：由 2～3 层扁平细胞构成，细胞界限不清，胞核退化消失，染成嗜酸性均质透明状。ⅴ 角质层：由多层扁平的角质细胞构成，细胞完全角化，界限不清，无细胞核，染色呈嗜酸性均质状，浅表层细胞连接松散。

② 真皮：与表皮相连，分为浅部的乳头层（papillary layer）和深部的网织层（reticular layer）。ⅰ 乳头层：位于真皮的浅层，为疏松结缔组织，向表皮底部突出形成很多乳头状隆起，称为真皮乳头（dermal papilla）。乳头内含有丰富的毛细血管，部分乳头内可见触觉小体（Meissner's corpuscles or tactile corpuscle），为梭形结构。ⅱ 网织层：位于真皮的深层，较厚，为不规则致密结缔组织，含有粗大的胶原纤维束和弹性纤维，含有较多血管、

神经纤维和汗腺(sweat glands)。深层可见环层小体(Pacini's corpuscles),为圆形或椭圆形的浅粉红结构。

高倍:仔细观察表皮各层细胞形态和真皮中的触觉小体、环层小体和汗腺的结构。

① 触觉小体:位于表皮下方的真皮乳头层中,呈梭形。触觉小体中可见深蓝色的扁平细胞核以及环层盘绕的淡粉色结构。

② 环层小体:位于真皮网织层内,可见同心圆形或椭圆形的淡红色结构,即为环层小体。多为环层小体横断面,位于中央的红色的点状为无髓神经纤维横截面,周围由数十层扁平细胞以同心圆的方式排列,外有结缔组织被囊。

③ 汗腺:分为分泌部(secretory apparatus)和导管部(duct apparatus)。分泌部管径较粗,由单层矮柱状或锥体形的腺细胞构成,胞质染色浅;导管部管径较细,由两层小立方细胞构成,胞质嗜碱性。

(3) 观察要点:区分表皮各层及真皮各层;观察触觉小体、环层小体、汗腺等结构。

2. 体皮 (Skin: body) (彩图 47)

(1) 取材和染色:体皮,HE 染色。

(2) 观察:

肉眼:可见染成紫色的一层为表皮,与掌皮相比较薄;染成粉红色的为真皮和皮下组织部分。

低倍:染成深紫色的一层为表皮,下方染成粉红色的组织为真皮和皮下组织。体皮为薄皮肤,表皮部分较薄,光镜下分为四层结构,由深部到表层分别为:基底层、棘层、颗粒层和角质层,无透明层,每一层的细胞结构与掌皮相似,但细胞层数少。真皮结构同掌皮。

高倍:仔细观察表皮各层细胞形态。

(3) 观察要点:区分表皮的各层结构,同掌皮比较。

3. 头皮(Skin: head) (彩图 48)

(1) 取材和染色:头皮,HE 染色。

(2) 观察:

肉眼:切片上染色较深的一面为表皮,染色较浅的一面为真皮和皮下组织,真皮中可见深紫色的结构为毛囊,部分毛囊中可见毛根。

低倍:

① 表皮:层次结构同体皮;

② 真皮:结构同体皮,内有毛根、毛囊(hair follicle)、立毛肌(arrector pili muscle)、皮脂腺(sebaceous gland)、汗腺等结构。毛根是毛发在皮肤内的结构,包绕在毛根周围的结构为毛囊,毛囊与表皮相连续,末端膨大为毛球(hair bulb)。立毛肌位于毛囊和皮肤成钝角的一侧,为红色的平滑肌束,连接毛囊与真皮乳头层。毛囊与立毛肌之间可见皮脂腺,为浅染的细胞团。

高倍:仔细观察真皮内毛囊和皮脂腺的结构。

① 毛囊：与表皮相延续，为复层上皮，染色深；毛囊的根部膨大成毛球，基底部有结缔组织突入，形成毛乳头(hair papilla)。

② 皮脂腺：腺细胞底部胞质嗜碱性，顶部胞质染色淡，细胞核位于中央，嗜碱性。

(3) 观察要点：毛囊、立毛肌、皮脂腺等。

三、思考题

1. 光镜下如何区分厚皮肤和薄皮肤？

2. 光镜下如何区分汗腺的分泌部与导管部？

（张昕昕，黄少萍）

Chapter 10
Skin

Ⅰ. Experiment purpose

1. To master the general structures of the epidermis and the dermis.
2. Familiarity with the characters of the hair, sebaceous glands and sweat glands.

Ⅱ. Experiment contents

1. Skin: palm (Figs. 43-46)

(1) Material and staining: Skin of palm, HE staining.

(2) Observe:

By eyes: The dark purple part is the epidermis and the pink part is the dermis and subcutaneous tissue.

Lower power lens: The dark purple part is the epidermis and the lower part is the dermis and subcutaneous tissue which are stained pink.

① Epidermis: The epidermis consists mainly of a stratified squamous keratinized epithelium. The skin of palm is thick skin, 5 epidermal layers are distinguishable under the microscopy, from deeper to surface, respectively, are stratum basale, stratum spinosum, stratum granulosum, stratum lucidum and stratum corneum. i Stratum basale: The stratum basale consists of a single layer of basophilic columnar or cuboidal cells, nuclei of these cells are ovoid and stained dark. ii Stratum spinosum: The stratum spinosum comprises 4-10 layers of large, polygonal cells, they have basophilic cytoplasm and large nuclei. iii Stratum granulosum: The stratum granulosum consists of 3-5 layers of diamond-shaped cells filled with dark-blue granules, the nuclei are almost disappear. iv Stratum lucidum: The stratum lucidum is a homogeneous, acidophilic and translucent band of 2-3 layers of flattened cells, whose nuclei and intercellular borders are not visible. v Stratum corneum: The stratum corneum consists of many layers of horny cells, they are completely keratinocytes, enucleate cells, and stained homogeneous acidophilic, the intercellular borders are invisible, and superficial cells are unconsolidated.

② Dermis: The dermis is joined to the epidermis, and consists the upper papillary layer and the lower reticular layer. i Papillary layer: The papillary layer lies beneath the epidermis, and is composed of loose connective tissue, it projects dermal papillae to the epidermal ridges, and there are many capillaries in the dermal papilla and some Meissner's corpuscles (tactile corpuscle), which are diamond-shaped. ii Reticular layer: The reticular layer, deep to the papillary layer, is a thicker layer of irregular dense connective tissue. This layer contains thick collagen fibers, elastic fibers, many blood vessels, nerve fibers and sweat glands. The reticular layer also contains Pacini's corpuscles, which are pink, circular or ovoid structures.

Higher power lens: Observe the structures of each layer of the epidermis, and the Meissner's corpuscles, the Pacini's corpuscles and the sweat glands in the dermis.

① Meissner's corpuscles: The Meissner's corpuscle is diamond-shaped, and located at the papillary layer of the dermis. Dark-blue, flattened nuclei and coiled, pink structures can be seen in the Meissner's corpuscles.

② Pacini's corpuscles: The Pacini's corpuscle is concentric circular or ovoid, pink structures, and located at the reticular layer of the dermis. The Pacini's corpuscles are mostly transverse section, in the center, a red-staining spot is the cross section of unmyelinated nerve fiber, encapsulate with about 10 layers of concentric circular, flattened cells.

③ Sweat glands: The sweat gland comprises the secretory apparatus and the duct apparatus. The lumen of the secretory apparatus is wider, and composed of a single layer of short columnar or pyramidal secretory cells, which are stained light. The wall of the duct is composed of stratified cuboidal epithelium, the cells that line the duct are smaller and stain darker.

(3) Observation key points: Five layers of the epidermis, two layers of the dermis, the Meissner's corpuscles, the Pacini's corpuscles, the sweat glands.

2. Skin: body (Fig. 47)

(1) Material and staining: Skin of body, HE staining.

(2) Observe:

By eyes: The dark purple part is the epidermis which is thinner than that of skin of palm, and the pink part is the dermis and subcutaneous tissue.

Lower power lens: The dark purple part is the epidermis and the lower part is the dermis and subcutaneous tissue which are stained pink. The skin of body is thin skin, the epidermis is thinner, and comprises 4 layers, from deeper to surface, respectively, are stratum basale, stratum spinosum, stratum granulosum, and stratum corneum, without stratum lucidum. The structure of each layer is similar to which of thick skin, yet with fewer layers of cells. The structure of the dermis is similar to that of thick skin.

Higher power lens: Observe the structures of every layer of the epidermis.

(3) Observation key points: the structure of each layer in the epidermis, and compare it with that of thick skin.

3. Skin: head (Fig. 48)

(1) Material and staining: Skin of head, HE staining.

(2) Observe:

By eyes: The dark purple part is the epidermis and the pink part is the dermis and subcutaneous tissue. Hair follicles can be seen in the dermis which are stained dark purple, hair roots can be seen in some hair follicles.

Lower power lens:

① Epidermis: The structure is the same as that of skin of body.

② Dermis: The structure is the same as that of skin of body, yet hair root, hair follicles, arrector pili muscle, sebaceous gland and sweat gland can also be seen in the dermis. The hair root is the part of hair inside the skin, encircled the hair root is the hair follicle, the follicles has a bulbous terminal called the hair bulb. The arrector pili muscle comprises smooth muscle cells, and is located at the obtuse angle connecting the hair follicles and the dermal papilla. Between the hair follicles and the arrector pili muscles are the sebaceous glands which are stained light.

Higher power lens: Observe the structure of the hair follicles and the sebaceous glands in the dermis.

① Hair follicles: The deep-stained hair follicle is the extension of the epidermis, which is stratified epithelium. The hair follicles has a bulbous terminal called the hair bulb, connective tissues called the hair papilla stick into the hair bulb.

② Sebaceous glands: The cytoplasm at the bottom part of glandular cell is basophilic, while the upper part is stained light, the nucleus is basophilic, located in center stained blue.

(3) Observation key points: hair follicles, arrector pili muscle, sebaceous gland.

III. Questions

1. How to distinguish the thick skin and the thin skin under the light microscopy?

2. How to distinguish the secretory apparatus and the duct apparatus of the sweat gland under the light microscopy?

(Zhang Xinxin, Huang Shaoping)

第十一章
消 化 管

一、实验目的

1. 掌握消化管壁的一般结构。

2. 掌握各段消化管壁的结构特点及区别。

二、实验内容

1. 食管（Esophagus）（彩图 49）

(1) 取材和染色：食管，HE 染色。

(2) 观察：

肉眼：可见圆形的食管横断面，管腔不规则，为食管壁的黏膜层和黏膜下层向管腔突起形成。腔面染成紫蓝色的结构为黏膜上皮。

低倍：由内向外依次观察管壁的四层结构。

① 黏膜（mucosa）：上皮为未角化的复层扁平上皮，上皮下方的固有层（lamina propria）为结缔组织，固有层外是黏膜肌层（muscularis mucosa），为纵行平滑肌，在食管横切面上表现为平滑肌的纵切面。

② 黏膜下层（submucosa）：为疏松结缔组织，内含丰富的黏液性食管腺（esophageal gland）。

③ 肌层（muscularis）：较厚，为内环肌和外纵肌。

④ 外膜（adventitia）：为疏松结缔组织，是纤维膜。

高倍：

① 仔细观察肌层属于哪种肌纤维，以此判断切片为食管上段、中段还是下段。

② 观察黏液性食管腺细胞的特征：细胞锥体形或柱状，细胞核扁平，位于细胞基底部，底部胞质弱嗜碱性，顶部胞质染色淡，呈空泡状。

(3) 观察要点：区分各层的结构，观察食管肌层的肌细胞种类、黏液性食管腺等。

2. 胃（Stomach）（彩图 50～51）

（1）取材和染色：胃底，HE 染色。

（2）观察：

肉眼：可见切成条状的胃底组织，凹凸不平的一面为胃内壁黏膜，光滑的一面为胃外壁浆膜，中间红色较厚部分为肌层。

低倍：

① 黏膜：ⅰ 胃壁黏膜上皮为单层柱状上皮，上皮向固有层内凹陷，形成胃小凹（gastric pit）。ⅱ 固有层内含有大量胃底腺（fundic gland or gastric gland）和少量结缔组织，胃底腺开口于胃小凹底部。切片中，胃底腺常被切成圆形或椭圆形断面，分为颈部、体部和底部三部分，底部嗜碱性，颈部嗜酸性。ⅲ 黏膜肌层为内环、外纵两层平滑肌。

② 黏膜下层：为疏松结缔组织。

③ 肌层：厚，分为内斜、中环、外纵三层平滑肌，切片上三层分界不明显。

④ 外膜：为结缔组织外被覆一层间皮构成，为浆膜（serosa）结构。

高倍：仔细观察黏膜上皮细胞和胃底腺细胞的形态。

① 黏膜上皮的单层柱状上皮细胞排列整齐，胞核椭圆形位于基底部，顶部胞质透亮呈空泡状。

② 主细胞（chief cell）多见于胃底腺的体部和底部，细胞呈柱状，核圆形，位于细胞基底部，胞质嗜碱性，切片中常呈空泡状。壁细胞（parietal cell）主要位于腺体的体部和颈部，胞体大，呈圆形或锥体形，核圆，居中，胞质强嗜酸性。颈黏液细胞（mucous neck cell）位于腺体颈部，数量少，不易找到，常呈楔形夹杂在其他细胞之间，胞核扁平，位于细胞基底部，胞质染色淡。

（3）观察要点：区分各层结构，辨认胃小凹、胃腺的主细胞、壁细胞等。

3. 空肠（Jejunum）（彩图 52～53，58～60）

（1）取材和染色：空肠，HE 染色。

（2）观察：

肉眼：切片上可见有褶皱的一面，为空肠的腔面，褶皱为环形皱襞（plicae circulares）；靠近较光滑的一面可见红色条带，为肌层。

低倍：黏膜与黏膜下层的结缔组织共同向管腔突出构成皱襞。皱襞上可见许多长指状突起，为小肠绒毛（intestinal villus），绒毛为固有层的结缔组织和小肠上皮共同向管腔突出形成。绒毛根部的上皮向固有层内凹陷，形成小肠腺（small intestinal gland），固有层内还可见孤立淋巴小结。固有层下的黏膜肌层薄，为内环、外纵两层平滑肌。黏膜下层由疏松结缔组织构成，有时可见黏膜下神经丛（submucosal plexus）。肌层分为内环、外纵两层平滑肌，两层之间可见肌间神经丛（myenteric nerve plexus），外膜为浆膜。

高倍：仔细观察小肠绒毛、小肠腺和肌间神经丛的结构。

① 小肠绒毛：小肠绒毛由小肠上皮和固有层的结缔组织共同向管腔突出形成。上皮

细胞主要由吸收细胞和杯状细胞构成，吸收细胞为柱状，胞核为椭圆形，位于细胞基底部，胞质嗜酸性。细胞游离面可见模糊的粉红色条带，为纹状缘(striated border)；杯状细胞夹杂在吸收细胞之间，形似高脚杯，胞核呈扁圆形或倒三角形，位于基底部，胞质顶部膨大呈空泡状。绒毛的固有层中可见中央乳糜管(central lacteal)、平滑肌和毛细血管，中央乳糜管位于轴心，管壁由内皮构成，切片中常呈压缩状态，故不明显(彩图 58)。

② 小肠腺：小肠腺为小肠黏膜上皮向固有层内凹陷形成，上皮细胞除了柱状细胞和杯状细胞外，在小肠腺的底部还可见到潘氏细胞(Paneth cell)，常三五成群聚集，锥体形，胞核顶部充满粗大的嗜酸性颗粒。

③ 肌间神经丛：位于内环肌与外纵肌之间，神经细胞较大，成群分布，细胞分界不清，胞核染色浅，核仁大而明显；胞质染色浅，可见蓝色细颗粒状、均匀分布的尼氏体(彩图 59)。黏膜下神经丛(彩图 60)和肌间神经丛结构基本相同。

(3) 观察要点：区分各层，观察小肠绒毛、小肠腺、纹状缘、杯状细胞、潘氏细胞、肌间神经丛、孤立淋巴小结。

4. 回肠 (Ileum)(彩图 54，58～60)

(1) 取材和染色：回肠，HE 染色。

(2) 观察：

肉眼：切片上可见有褶皱的一面，为回肠的腔面，褶皱为环形皱襞(plicae circulares)；靠近较光滑的一面可见红色条带，为肌层。

低倍：结构同空肠基本相同。小肠绒毛呈阔叶状，小肠腺潘氏细胞较少，固有层内有半圈集合淋巴小结(注意与空肠相区别)。

高倍：结构同空肠基本相同。

(3) 观察要点：与空肠相同。

5. 结肠 (Colon)(彩图 55～56)

(1) 取材和染色：结肠，HE 染色。

(2) 观察：

肉眼：被切成长条状组织，染成紫色的部分为黏膜，染成红色的部分为肌层。

低倍：同小肠相比较：结肠无绒毛，大肠腺发达，富含杯状细胞。大肠腺直而长，排列紧密，切片中可见大肠腺的不同断面。固有层内淋巴组织丰富。肌层为内环、外纵两层平滑肌，外膜为结缔组织，可见较多脂肪细胞。

高倍：同小肠相比较：黏膜上皮杯状细胞较多，腺上皮主要为杯状细胞，无潘氏细胞。

(3) 观察要点：区分各层，观察黏膜上皮、大肠腺。

6. 阑尾 (Appendix)(彩图 57)

(1) 取材和染色：阑尾，HE 染色。

(2) 观察：

肉眼:可见阑尾的横切面,为圆形管腔,管腔较小。

低倍:阑尾无绒毛,上皮及大肠腺与结肠类似,但肠腺短而少。固有层内淋巴组织丰富,形成一圈集合淋巴小结,并伸入黏膜下层,故黏膜肌层不完整。肌层薄,分为内环、外纵两层,外膜为浆膜。

高倍:仔细观察阑尾的上皮与大肠腺。

(3) 观察要点:区分各层,观察黏膜上皮、大肠腺、固有层淋巴组织。

三、思考题

1. 消化管壁的一般结构是什么?
2. 食管的结构特点是什么? 胃的结构特点是什么? 试述壁细胞的结构和功能。
3. 光镜下如何区分空肠、回肠与阑尾?

(张昕昕,黄少萍)

Chapter 11
Digestive Tract

Ⅰ. Experiment purpose

1. To master the general structures of the digestive tracts.

2. To master the key points of each part of the digestive tract, and tell the differences between them.

Ⅱ. Experiment contents

1. Esophagus (Fig. 49)

(1) Material and staining: Esophagus, HE staining.

(2) Observe:

By eyes: Transverse section of the esophagus can be seen. The lumen is irregular because of the protrusion of the mucosa and the submucosa. The surface of the lumen is the mucosa epithelium, which is stained purple.

Lower power lens: From the inner to the outer part, the wall can be divided into four layer.

① The epithelium is the nonkeratinized stratified squamous epithelium. Under the epithelium is connective tissue, which is called the lamina propria, the outer part is the muscularis mucosa which is a single layer of smooth muscle cells arranged in the same direction as the tract.

② The submucosa is loose connective tissue, and rich in mucous esophageal gland.

③ The muscularis is thick and can be divided into the inner circular and external longitudinal layer.

④ The adventitia is composed of loose connective tissue.

Higher power lens:

① Observe the muscularis carefully, tell which kind of muscle cell it belongs to, and then you will know which part of the esophagus the section belongs to.

② The cells of the mucous esophageal gland are pyramidal or columnar, the flattened nuclei locate at the bottom part of the cells, the cytoplasm at the bottom part is basophilic, and the upper part is stained light.

(3) Observation key points: Distinguish the four layers, observe the muscularis, the mucous esophagus gland.

2. Stomach (Figs. 50-51)

(1) Material and staining: Stomach, HE staining.

(2) Observe:

By eyes: The stripped tissue is the stomach, the irregular surface is the mucosa, and the smooth surface is the adventitia, the red part is the muscularis.

Lower power lens:

① The mucosa: ⅰ epithelium is the simple columnar epithelium, it invaginates into the lamina propria and forms the gastric pits.

ⅱ The lamina propria is composed of many fundic or gastric glands and connective tissues, there are openings of the gastric glands on the bottom of the gastric pits. The gastric glands are usually shown as circular or ovoid sections, and can be divided into three parts: neck, body and bottom, the bottom part is basophilic and the neck part is eosinophil.

ⅲ Outside the gastric glands there are the inner circular and external longitudinal muscularis mucosa.

② The submucosa is composed of loose connective tissue.

③ The muscularis is thick and include three layers of muscle cells according different directions: the inner oblique layer, the middle circular layer and the outer longitudinal layer.

④ The adventitia comprises connective tissue coating mesothelium, this structure is called the serosa.

Higher power lens: Observe the cells of the mucosa epithelium and gastric glands.

① The nuclei of the aligned columnar cells are at the bottom part, and the cytoplasm is at the upper part and stained light.

② The columnar chief cells are at the body and bottom part of the gastric glands, the nuclei are circular and at the basal part, the cytoplasm is light basophilic. The parietal cells are at the body and neck part of the gastric glands, the cells are large and in circular or pyramidal shaped, the nuclei are round and in the center, the cytoplasm is deep eosinophil. The mucous neck cells are at the neck part of the gastric glands, they are difficult to find because of the small quantity. The cells are wedge-shaped and intersperse between other cells. The flattened nuclei locate at the basal part, and the cytoplasm is stained light.

(3) Observation key points: Distinguish the four layers; observe the gastric glands (the chief cells, the parietal cells), the gastric pits.

3. Jejunum (Figs. 52-53, 58-60)

(1) Material and staining: Jejunum, HE staining.

(2) Observe:

By eyes: The irregular surface of the section is the inner surface, and you can see the plicae circulares. Near the regular surface we can see the red muscularis.

Lower power lens: The plicae circulares is composed of mucosa and submucosa and fingerlike mucosal projections into the lumen to form many intestinal villi, which are composed of lamina propria and mucosa. The mucosa epithelium also extends into the lamina propria below the bases of the villi to form small intestinal glands. Solitary lymphoid nodule can be seen in the lamina propria. Outside the lamina propria there are the inner circular and external longitudinal muscularis mucosa. The submucosa comprises loose connective tissue, submucosal nerve plexus can be seen in this layer. The muscularis can be divided into internal circular layer and the outer longitudinal layer, and between these two layers there are some myenteric nerve plexus. The adventitia is the serosa.

Higher power lens: Observe the structure of the intestinal villi, the intestinal glands and the myenteric nerve plexus.

① Intestinal villus: The intestinal epithelium and the lamina propria project into the lumen to form the intestinal villus. The epithelium consists of absorptive cells and goblet cells. The absorptive cells are columnar, the ovoid nuclei are located at the basal part, the cytoplasm is eosinophil, and in the free surface there is a layer of striated border which is stained pink. There are goblet cells between the absorptive cells, the oblate or inverted triangular-shaped nuclei are located near the basal part of the cell, and the apical part of these cells is vacuolar. The lamina propria core of each villus consists of loose connective tissue and contains a central lacteal, smooth muscle cells and capillaries. The central lacteal locates on the axis, whose wall is composed of endothelium, it is often compressed and difficult to observe.

② Small intestinal gland: The mucosa epithelium extends into the lamina propria below the bases of the villi to form intestinal glands. Besides the columnar cells and the goblet cells, there are also Paneth cells in the bottom of the intestinal gland, the cells are pyramidal, and gather in groups, above the nuclei, coarse acidophil granules can be seen in the cytoplasm.

③ Myenteric nerve plexus: Between the internal circular layer and the outer longitudinal layer muscularis, there are myenteric nerve plexus. The neuron is large and in groups, the nucleus is stained light, and the nucleolus is large and clear, the cytoplasm is stained light and contains many blue granules called Nissl bodies (Fig. 59). The structure of the submucosal plexus (Fig. 60) is similar to that of the myenteric nerve plexus.

(3) Observation key points: intestinal villus, small intestinal gland, myenteric nerve plexus, striated border, goblet cell, Paneth cell, myenteric nerve plexus, solitary lymphoid nodule.

4. Ileum (Figs. 54, 58-60)

(1) Material and staining: Ileum, HE staining.

(2) Observe:

By eyes: The irregular surface of the section is the inner surface, and you can see the plicae circulares. Near the regular surface we can see the red muscularis.

Lower power lens: Same as the jejunum. Distinguish it from the jejunum.

Higher power lens: Same as the jejunum. Distinguish it from the jejunum.

(3) Observation key points: Same as the jejunum.

5. Colon (Figs. 55-56)

(1) Material and staining: Colon, HE staining.

(2) Observe:

By eyes: The stripped tissue is colon, mucosa is stained purple, and the muscularis is stained red.

Lower power lens: Compared with the small intestine, the colon has no villus, the lamina propria is rich in lymphatic tissues and large intestine gland, which is straight and long. The muscularis can be divided into internal circular layer and the outer longitudinal layer. The adventitia is composed of connective tissue, and contains many adipose cells.

Higher power lens: Compared with the small intestine, the mucosa epithelium of the colon contains more goblet cells, the epithelium of the gland also contains many goblet cells, and no Paneth cell.

(3) Observation key points: mucosa epithelium, large intestine gland.

6. Appendix (Fig. 57)

(1) Material and staining: Appendix, HE staining.

(2) Observe:

By eyes: The round tissue is the cross section of appendix, the lumen is round and small.

Lower power lens: The appendix has no villus. The epithelium and large intestine gland are similar to that of the colon, while the gland is shorter. Many lymphatic nodules can be seen in the lamina propria, and extend to the submucosa. The muscularis mucosa is discontinuous. The thin muscularis can be divided into internal circular layer and the outer longitudinal layer. The adventitia is serosa.

Higher power lens: Observe the epithelium and large intestine gland of the appendix.

(3) Observation key points: mucosa epithelium, large intestine gland, lymphatic tissue in the lamina propria.

III. Questions

1. What are the general characters of the digestive tract?

2. What are the structural features of the esophagus? What are the structural characters of the stomach? Describe the structure and function of the parietal cells.

3. How to distinguish the jejunum, the ileum and the appendix under the light microscopy?

(Zhang Xinxin, Huang Shaoping)

第十二章
消　化　腺

一、实验目的

1. 熟悉浆液性腺泡、黏液性腺泡、混合性腺泡的结构特点。
2. 掌握胰腺的结构及功能。
3. 掌握肝脏的基本结构及功能。
4. 掌握肝细胞和肝血窦的光、电镜结构。

二、实验内容

1. 胰腺（Pancreas）（彩图 61～63）

（1）取材与染色：胰腺，HE 染色。

（2）观察：

肉眼：紫红色的组织为胰腺，其间可见散在的浅染区域，即胰岛。

低倍：粉红色的结缔组织被膜伸入实质，将胰腺分隔成许多小叶。小叶内可见大量浆液性腺泡，染成紫红色，以及散在的大小不等的细胞团，即胰岛，染色较浅。

高倍：① 胰腺腺泡细胞锥体形，上部胞质中含有较多的酶原颗粒，故染成紫红色。基部胞质因含大量粗面内质网而染成紫蓝色。

② 腺泡腔中，可见泡心细胞（由闰管上皮细胞延伸进腺泡腔形成），核圆形或卵圆形，胞质淡。

③ 闰管由单层扁平或立方上皮围成，与腺泡相连；胰腺无纹状管，小叶内导管由单层立方上皮组成，小叶间导管壁由单层柱状上皮组成。

④ 胰岛呈大小不等、形状不规则的细胞团，染色淡，分散在腺泡之间。构成胰岛的四种细胞 HE 染色下不能区分，胰岛内可见毛细血管。

（3）观察要点：胰腺小叶、腺泡、泡心细胞、小叶间导管、闰管、胰岛等。

2. 肝脏（Live）（彩图 64～67）

（1）取材与染色：肝脏，HE 染色。

(2) 观察:

肉眼:可见染成红色的实质性肝脏组织。

低倍:表面为红色的致密结缔组织被膜,被膜上被覆有单层扁平上皮(间皮)。正常人肝小叶周围结缔组织少,故肝小叶的范围不清楚。猪肝中,因为结缔组织较多,故肝小叶结构较清楚。

① 小叶中央为中央静脉,形态不规则、管壁有肝血窦的开口,腔中有血细胞。

② 肝细胞单层排列成肝索,以中央静脉为中心向四周呈放射状排列。

③ 肝索之间为肝血窦。

④ 相邻肝小叶间的三角形或不规则形的结缔组织区域,称门管区,可见三种伴行的管道,即小叶间动脉、小叶间静脉、小叶间胆管。

⑤ 在小叶间结缔组织中,有时管腔较大、管壁较厚的静脉单独行走,为小叶下静脉。

高倍:① 中央静脉壁薄,腔面由单层内皮覆盖。

②肝索由单层的肝细胞组成。肝细胞体积较大,多边形,界限清楚,核圆,位于中央,染色淡,核膜清晰,可见双核。

③ 肝血窦壁为单层扁平上皮,核扁圆,胞质少,呈粉红色线状;窦腔可见肝巨噬细胞,体积较大且不规则,核呈卵圆形,染色较淡,胞质红色,血窦腔还可见各种血细胞。

④ 血窦壁上皮和肝细胞之间,可见狭小的区域,为窦周隙。

⑤ 门管区的小叶间胆管由单层立方上皮围成,核为圆或椭圆形,染色较深。小叶间动脉管径细,管壁较厚,由数层环行平滑肌围成。小叶间静脉腔大壁薄不规则,管壁由内皮、薄层结缔组织及少量平滑肌构成。

(3) 观察要点:辨认肝小叶界限,观察中央静脉、肝细胞、肝索、肝血窦、窦周隙、门管区及其三种管道,比较人肝与猪肝的差异。

3. 下颌下腺(Submandibular gland)(彩图 68)

(1) 取材与染色:下颌下腺,HE 染色。

(2) 观察:

肉眼:可见数个小叶,小叶中的淡染区为黏液性腺泡所在的部位。

低倍:结缔组织被膜伸入实质,将其分隔成许多小叶,小叶内可见腺泡和导管。导管染色较红而明显,可见少量结缔组织和血管。浆液性腺泡 HE 染色呈紫红色结构,粘液性腺泡为浅染结构。

高倍:腺泡可分为三类:

① 黏液性腺泡:细胞呈锥体形或立方形,核扁圆形,位于基底部,细胞着色为浅蓝色或呈空泡状。

② 浆液性腺泡:腺泡腔较小,腺细胞锥体形,核椭圆形,位于基部,顶部胞质含嗜酸性的内分泌颗粒,呈红色,基部胞质嗜碱性强,呈蓝紫色。

③ 混合性腺泡:常见黏液性腺泡一侧包有数个浆液性腺细胞,呈新月状,称浆半月。

导管可见四段:① 闰管:与腺泡直接相连,管壁由单层扁平或矮立方上皮组成。

② 分泌管:接于闰管之后,管径明显增粗,管壁为单层高柱状上皮细胞,胞质嗜酸性,呈红色,细胞基部纵纹不明显。

③ 小叶内导管:为分泌管之后的管道,管壁稍细于分泌管,由矮柱状上皮细胞组成,胞质染色较浅。

④ 小叶间导管:行走于小叶间结缔组织中,管壁为假复层柱状上皮,常与血管、神经伴行。

(3) 观察要点:三种腺泡及四种管道。

三、思考题

1. 光镜下可见到肝小叶的哪些结构?

2. 在肝门管区,如何区分小叶间动脉、小叶间静脉、小叶间胆管?

3. 在切片上如何区分浆液性腺泡和黏液性腺泡?

(黄少萍,朱丽娟)

Chapter 12
Digestive Gland

Ⅰ. Experiment purpose

1. Be familiar with the structural characteristics of serous, mucinous and mixed acini.
2. Master the structure and function of the pancreas.
3. Master the fundamental structure of the liver lobules and the portal area.
4. Master the light and electron microscopic structures of the hepatocyte and hepatic sinusoid.

Ⅱ. Experiment contents

1. Pancreas (Figs. 61-63)

(1) Materials: Pancreas, HE staining.

(2) Observe:

By eyes: The parenchyma is stained in purple red colour with some light staining areas named as islets of Langerhans.

Lower power lens: The pancreas is divided by connective tissue into some lobules. A lobule mainly consists of serous acinus. Some lobules also contain pancreatic islets of Langerhans with different volumes. The serous acinus is stained in purple red color whereas the pancreatic islets of Langerhans are stained palely, scattered among pancreatic serous acini. The pancreatic islets of Langerhans are vary widely in the size.

Higher power lens:

① Serous acinus is made up of a layer of pyramidal cells with round nuclei situated toward the base of the cells. The subnuclear cytoplasm of the cell is strong basophilic.

② A few round nuclei are present in the lumen of the serous acinus, these are the nuclei of the centroacinar cells, which derived from the intercalated duct.

③ The interlobular ducts are in the septa between the lobules. They are lined with simple columnar epithelium and surround by connective tissue. The septum also contains blood vessels.

④ The pancreatic islets of Langerhans are a pale-staining cluster of cells, are surrounded by more intensely stained pancreatic acini. It is not practical to identify the several cell types found in the HE stain specimens.

(3) Observation key points: lobule, serous acinus, centroacinar cell, intercalated duct, interlobular duct, pancreatic islets of Langerhans, etc.

2. Liver (Figs. 64–67)

(1) Materials: Liver, HE staining.

(2) Observe:

By eyes: The liver tissue is stained in red colour.

Lower power lens: The parenchyma of a liver is divided by connective tissue into many polygonal structures, namely hepatic lobules. In normal human, the lobule's border is not clear because of less connective tissue. In pig, the border of hepatic lobule is clear because of more connective tissue.

① A blood vessel with a large lumen locates in the center of the lobule, is the central vein.

② The hepatocytes are radially arranged around the central vein forming many hepatocyte cords.

③ The spaces between the hepatocyte cords are liver sinusoids. The wall of the center vein is disrupted by the opening of the hepatic sinusoids.

④ The portal areas are the connective tissue between the corners of several lobules, in which there are three kinds of vessels: interlobular vein, interlobular artery, and interlobular bile duct.

⑤ In the interlobular connective tissue, sometimes, vein with larger lumen and thicker wall is the sublobular vein, it presents lonely.

Higher power lens:

① Central vein has a very thin wall, its lumen surface is covered by the endothelium.

② Hepatocyte is large polygonal cell, the nuclear is round locating in the center of the cell, and the cytoplasm is rich, eosinophilic with fine basophilic granules. Hepatocytes are radially arranged to form many single layer of cell cords.

③ Sinusoid is an irregular space located the between the adjacent hepatic plates. It is lined with simple endothelial cells.

④ Disse space, is the space between the hepatocytes and the endothelial cells of the sinusoid.

⑤ Portal area: there are three kinds of vessels: interlobular vein, interlobular artery, and interlobular bile duct. The lumen of the interlobular artery is small in diameter with a thick wall consisting of several circular smooth muscles. The lumen of the interlobular vein is large in diameter with an irregular outline and a very thin wall. The interlobular bile duct has a small round lumen lined by a layer of cuboidal cells.

(3) Observation key points: Hepatic lobules, central vein, hepatocytes, hepatic cords, Disse space, Portal area and three kinds of vessels in this area. Compare the differences between the human liver and the pig liver.

3. Submandibular gland (Fig. 68)

(1) Materials: Submandibular gland, HE staining.

(2) Observe:

By eyes: The parenchyma which stained deeply is separated into lobules by the connective tissue stained paler.

Lower power lens: The septa of the lobules contains loose connective tissue, blood vessels and ducts. Lobule contains the serous, mucous and mixed acinus. The serous acinus are stained with HE as purple red structures; the mucous acinus as pale structures.

Higher power lens: To distinguish three types of the acinus.

① Mucous acinus: Cytoplasm of the serous cells is clearly purple red whereas the cytoplasm of the mucous cells appears as empty. This is results of losing the mucus in cytoplasm during the preparation of routine HE section.

② Serous acinus: The nuclei of serous cells are oval or spherical located at the basal part of the cells. The basal cytoplasm of serous cell is strong stained with hematoxylin. The nuclei of the mucous cells often appear flattened and are pressed against the base of the cell.

③ Mixed acinus: Some of the serous cells form a cap at the end of the mucous acinus, this cap consisting of serous cells is called demilune. The mucous acinus with a demilune is called a mixed acinus (alveolus).

The ducts include 4 segments:

① Intercalated ducts: directly attached to the acinus, its surface is covered by a simple squamous or cuboidal epithelium.

② Secretory duct: diameter of the duct was significantly increased. Its wall was covered by a layer of high columnar epithelial cells with eosinophilic cytoplasm and no obvious longitudinal striation at the base of the cell.

③ Intralobular duct: the duct is composed of short columnar epithelial cells with lighter staining in cytoplasm.

④ Interlobular catheter: it locates in the interlobular connective tissue, and the lumen surface is covered by pseudostratified columnar epithelium, always companied by blood vessels and nerves.

(3) Observation key points: Serous acinus, mucous acinus, mixed acinus, striated ducts, and so on.

Ⅲ. Questions

1. What structures of hepatic lobules can be seen under the light microscope?
2. In the portal area of liver, how to distinguish the interlobular artery, interlobular vein, interlobular bile duct?
3. How to distinguish the serous acinus from the mucous acinus?

(Huang Shaoping, Zhu Lijuan)

第十三章
呼 吸 系 统

一、实验目的

1. 掌握气管的组织结构特点。

2. 掌握支气管结构特点及其变化规律;掌握肺呼吸部各部的结构特点。

二、实验内容

1.气管(Trachea)(彩图 4)

(1) 取材和染色:气管,HE 染色。

(2) 观察:

肉眼:可见圆形气管横切面,壁中的紫蓝色结构为透明软骨。

低倍:由内向外依次分黏膜、黏膜下层、外膜三层结构。

① 黏膜最内面的部分为假复层纤毛柱状上皮,上皮下为固有层结缔组织,因弹性纤维较多故染色较红。

② 黏膜下层与固有层之间无明显的界限,黏膜下层可见混合性腺体。

③ 外膜较厚,含透明软骨环和结缔组织。

高倍:① 黏膜上皮为假复层纤毛柱状上皮,含较多杯状细胞。固有层中有大量弹性纤维的横断面,呈红色小点。此弹性纤维可作为固有层和黏膜下层的分界。

② 黏膜下层中的腺体为混合腺,可见浆液性、黏液性、混合性三种腺泡。

③ 外膜的结缔组织中可见“C 形”的透明软骨环,软骨环的背侧部分可见平滑肌。

(3) 观察要点:分清三层结构,观察假复层纤毛柱状上皮、固有层、腺体、透明软骨环等结构。

2. 肺(Lung)(彩图 69~72)

(1) 取材和染色:肺,HE 染色。

(2) 观察:

肉眼：可见染色为粉红色的海绵样组织。

低倍：肺外表面被覆浆膜，为胸膜脏层（单层扁平上皮）。肺实质主要由各级支气管、大量的肺泡和毛细血管组成。

① 切片中较大的管子为小支气管。管壁完整、较厚，分为三层：黏膜的上皮为假复层纤毛柱状上皮，杯状细胞较少；固有层薄；有不完整的环行平滑肌。黏膜下层内有腺体。外膜内含断续的透明软骨片。

② 细支气管管径较小，上皮渐变为单层纤毛柱状，杯状细胞更少或消失；环行平滑肌相对增多；腺体和软骨片更少或消失。

③ 终末细支气管仅由一层黏膜组成，上皮为单层柱状上皮，无杯状细胞；固有层很薄不明显；有完整的环行平滑肌；无腺体和软骨。

④ 呼吸性细支气管管壁更薄，有少量肺泡开口故不完整，上皮为单层立方上皮，下有少量结缔组织和平滑肌。

⑤ 肺泡管有大量肺泡开口，故残存管壁少而形成结节性膨大：表面为单层立方上皮或单层扁平上皮、内含少量结缔组织和平滑肌。

⑥ 肺泡囊由几个肺泡的围成。

⑦ 肺泡呈半球形或球形，数量多，壁很薄。

高倍：①肺泡内表面被覆单层扁平上皮（Ⅰ型细胞），界限不清。②上皮下为少量结缔组织，富含毛细血管。肺泡Ⅰ型细胞和Ⅱ型细胞不要求区分。③肺泡腔内可见巨噬细胞（肺尘细胞）：胞体大、圆形或不规则形，核小深染，胞质内可见棕褐色、大小不一的吞噬颗粒（为吞噬的灰尘等）。

（3）观察要点：小支气管、细支气管、终末细支气管、呼吸性细支气管、肺泡管、肺泡囊、肺泡及尘细胞等，总结管壁结构的渐变过程。

三、思考题

1. 气管的结构特点是什么？
2. 如何区别肺内各级支气管？
3. 从气管到终末细支气管的各级管壁变化规律是什么？
4. 描述气血屏障的结构。

（纪红，黄少萍）

Chapter 13
Respiratory System

Ⅰ. Experiment purpose

1. Master the structures of the trachea.

2. Master the structures of the conduction portion and the respiratory portion in the lungs.

Ⅱ. Experiment contents

1. Trachea (Fig. 4)

(1) Materials: Trachea, HE staining.

(2) Observe:

By eyes: The circular structure is the transverse section of the trachea, the wall of the trachea contains the blue hyaline cartilage showed as ring-shaped.

Lower power lens: Distinguish the mucosa, submucosa and the adventitia from each other.

① Mucosa: The pseudostratified ciliated columnar epithelium which contains lots of goblet cells. The lamina propria is consisted of loose connective tissue.

② Submucosa: There is no clear boundary between the submucosa and lamina propria, mixed glands can be seen in the submucosa. There is no distinct boundary between the lamina propria and the submucosa.

③ Adventitia: This layer contains the C-shaped hyaline cartilage.

Higher power lens:

① The mucosa is covered with pseudostratified ciliated columnar epithelium. The epithelium contains a number of goblet cells, the lamina propria is made up of loose connective tissue which contains many small blood vessels and the glandular ducts.

② The submucosa is composed of loose connective tissue which contains numerous seromucous gland (mixed glands).

③ The adventitia is mainly composed of loose connective tissue and a piece of the C-shaped hyaline cartilage which is covered by a layer of dense connective tissue. At the dorsal region of the cartilage, you can find smooth muscle fibers.

(3) Observation key points: Distinguish the three layers, pseudostratified ciliated columnar epithelium, lamina propria, seromucous gland, C-shaped hyaline cartilage, and so on.

2. Lung (Figs. 69–72)

(1) Materials: Lung, HE stain.

(2) Observe:

By eyes: The specimen appears as a red honeycomb-like structure.

Lower power lens: Try to distinguish the conducting portion including the small bronchi, bronchioles and terminal bronchioles and the respiratory portion including the respiratory bronchioles, alveolar ducts, alveolar sacs and alveoli. Recognize them according to their diameters of the lumen and the structure of the walls. Identify the following structures in the section:

① Small bronchi: After entering the lungs, the bronchi subdivide repeatedly into small bronchi. They have a similar structure to that of the trachea. But as the diameter of bronchus becomes smaller, its wall becomes thinner, the number of goblet cells and glands gradually decreases and the C-shaped cartilaginous plates also become smaller and fewer. On the other hand, smooth muscles increase relatively between the lamina propria and submucosa.

② Bronchioles: The lumen is covered by the single ciliated columnar cells with fewer goblet cells. Glands and plates of hyaline cartilage become less and disappear. The circular smooth muscle layer become clearly.

③ Terminal bronchioles: Their wall mainly contain a layer of columnar epithelium and a continuous layer of circular smooth muscle fibers.

④ Respiratory bronchioles: The walls with a few alveoli are interrupted by few openings of the alveoli. The epithelium is low columnar or cuboidal. Beneath the epithelium a few of smooth muscle fibers surround it.

⑤ Alveolar ducts: The alveolar duct presents a very discontinuous wall with lots of openings of the alveoli. The remaining wall between the adjacent alveoli showed as the knobs — the epithelium is simple cuboidal or squamous.

⑥ Alveolar sacs: They are consist of groups of alveoli clustered around a common air space. Alveolar sacs have no walls.

⑦ Alveoli: the alveolus is a small thin-walled sac-like pocket. Higher power lens: Alveoli are the irregularly vesicular structure. Its wall is lined with simple squamous epithelium.

Higher power lens:

① Type I cells cannot be distinguished from type II cells.

② The alveolar wall containing numerous capillaries is called interalveolar septum.

③ Alveolar macrophages appear in the septa or in the lumen of the alveoli. These macrophages also are called dust cells after they have phagocytized dust. Dust cells contains particles of phagocytosed dust in their cytoplasm exhibiting black color.

(3) Observation key points: Distinguish the small bronchi, bronchioles and terminal bronchioles and the respiratory portion including the respiratory bronchioles, alveolar ducts, alveolar sacs and alveoli. Summarize the transitional changes of the conducting parts.

III. Questions

1. What are the structures of the trachea?
2. How to distinguish small bronchi, bronchioles and terminal bronchiole, respiratory bronchioles from each other?
3. What is transitional changes of structures from the trachea to terminal bronchiole?
4. Describe the components of the blood-air barriers.

(Ji Hong, Huang Shaoping)

第十四章
泌 尿 系 统

一、实验目的

1. 掌握肾单位的组成、肾小体的光镜结构。掌握近端小管曲部和远端小管上皮细胞的光镜结构特点。

2. 熟悉肾小管其余各段和集合管系的结构特点；熟悉球旁复合体的组成及功能。

3. 了解膀胱的组织结构。

二、实验内容

1. 肾（Kidney）（彩图 73～75）

（1）取材和染色：肾，HE 染色。

（2）观察：

肉眼：染色深的部分是皮质，染色浅的部分是髓质。髓质中，尖端很浅的部分为内带，靠近皮质略深的部分为外带。

低倍：表面结缔组织被膜的下方为皮质，有许多球形的肾小体和泌尿小管断面，多为近端小管曲部和远端小管曲部，管径粗细不等、形状不一。皮质内可见无肾小体而有直行管道的区域，称髓放线。髓放线之间有肾小体及肾小管的区域为皮质迷路。皮质内侧染色较浅的为髓质，内无肾小体而均为管子。皮质和髓质交界处，可见较大的小动、静脉，即弓形动、静脉。

高倍：

① 皮质

ⅰ 肾小体：皮质内的球形结构为肾小体，由血管球和肾小囊组成。血管球为一团毛细血管，内可见血细胞，结构较难分辨。肾小囊分脏、壁两层：脏层紧贴血管球的外面，为足细胞，不易分辨；壁层为单层扁平上皮。脏层和壁层之间的腔隙即肾小囊腔。

ⅱ 近端小管曲部：管腔较小而不规则，管壁较厚，上皮为单层立方或锥体形，核呈圆形，偏于基底部，胞质染色嗜酸性很强，红色。细胞界限不清楚，游离面可见刷状缘。

ⅲ 远端小管曲部：管腔较大，管壁较薄，上皮细胞较低，胞质染色较近端小管曲部浅。

ⅳ 致密斑：位于肾小体血管极处。远端小管在近肾小体血管极侧，其管壁上皮细胞呈柱状，核呈卵圆形，细胞排列紧密，称致密斑。入球微动脉和出球微动脉很难切到，不要求找。

② 髓质

ⅰ 近直小管：结构与曲部相似，管径比曲部细，管壁上皮的胞质染色较近曲小管上皮染色淡。

ⅱ 细段：管壁薄，为单层扁平上皮围成，核着色浅。注意与血管区别。

ⅲ 远直小管：管径较小，管壁上皮细胞胞质染色比近端小管直部更浅。

ⅳ 集合小管系：各段的管腔均较大，管壁上皮为单层立方或柱状，乳头管则呈高柱状。细胞界限清楚，核为圆形或卵圆形，深染，胞质清亮，浅染。

（3）观察要点：分清皮、髓质，观察肾小体、近端小管、远端小管、细段、致密斑和集合管等结构。

2. 膀胱（Bladder）（彩图 6）

（1）取材和染色：膀胱，HE 染色。

（2）观察：

肉眼：可见有空腔结构的组织，为膀胱。

低倍：从内向外分三层：黏膜、肌层和外膜。黏膜向膀胱腔突起形成皱襞，由上皮（变移上皮）和固有层组成。表层细胞大圆形或长方形，称盖细胞。上皮下方为固有层结缔组织。肌层：很厚，可见各种切面的平滑肌，排列不规则，故不必分层。外膜：是浆膜。

高倍：注意上皮细胞的形态。

（3）观察要点：膀胱分层，变移上皮的形态。

三、思考题

1. 试述肾单位的组织结构及其与功能的关系。
2. 试述肾小体的组织结构及其与功能的关系。
3. 在光镜下如何鉴别近端小官曲部和远端小管曲部？

（吴晓菁，黄少萍）

Chapter 14
Urinary system

Ⅰ. Experiment purpose

1. Master the structures of the renal corpuscle, proximal tubule and distal tubule under the light microscope.

2. Familiarity with the structures of the thin segment and the collecting tubules under the light microscopic.

3. Understand the structure of the bladder under the light microscope.

Ⅱ. Experiment contents

1. Kidney (Figs. 73-75)

(1) Materials: Kidney, HE staining.

(2) Observe:

By eyes: The cortex is stronger staining yet the medulla is lighter staining.

Lower power lens: The surface of the kidney is covered with a capsule composed of dense connective tissue. The parenchyma may be divided into an outer cortex and an inner medulla. The renal cortex is deeper-stained and consists mainly of renal corpuscles, proximal convoluted tubules and distal convoluted tubules. The renal medulla is paler-stained and there is no renal corpuscle. It is composed of a large number of different parts of renal tubules. Most of them are transverse section.

Higher power lens:

① Cortex: ⅰ Renal corpuscles: they are spherical, and consist of glomerulus and renal capsule. The glomerulus consists of a tuft of capillaries enveloped in the renal capsule. The renal capsule can be divided into parietal layer and visceral layer. The parietal layer of the capsule is simple squamous epithelium which is easy to identify. The visceral layer (podocytes) enveloping the capillaries of glomerulus is difficult to distinguish. The cavity between the two layers is the capsular space. ⅱ Proximal convoluted tubule: They are near the renal corpuscle. The lumen are lined by simple cuboidal or pyramidal cells, the wall of the tubules is thick and the lumen is relatively small and irregular. Their boundaries are obscure and cytoplasm is acidophil. Brush border on the free surface of these cells is not easy to be found, because it is usually destroyed during the preparation. ⅲ Distal convoluted tubule: The cross sections of the distal convoluted tubules are fewer than that of the proximal convoluted tubules. The lumen are lined by simple cuboidal epithelium with pale-stained cytoplasm. The lumen of the tubule is large and regular. The cellular boundaries are clearer than those of the proximal. ⅳ Epithelial cells of distal tubules near the vascular pole side transform to columnar, these calls are arranged closely to form the macula densa.

② Medulla: ⅰ Proximal straight tubules: Comparing to the proximal convoluted part, the straight tubule is similar to the convoluted part, but the diameter is smaller, the cytoplasmic of the tubular epithelial cell is lighter staining. ⅱ Thin segment: The wall of the tubule is consisted of simple squamous epithelium with pale nuclear. Differentiate the thin segment from the blood vessels. ⅲ Distal straight tubule: The diameter of the tube is small, and the cytoplasmic staining of the tubular epithelial cell is paler than that of the proximal straight tubule. ⅳ Collecting tubule: The lumen are larger, the epithelium of the tubule is a single layer of cubic or columnar cells or high columnar. The cell boundary is clearly, nuclear is round or ovoid, cytoplasm is pale staining.

(3) Observation key points: Identify the cortex and medulla, renal corpuscles, renal capsule, proximal convoluted tubules, distal convoluted tubules, thin segments and macula densa.

2. Bladder (Fig. 6)

(1) Materials: Bladder, HE staining.

(2) Observe:

By eyes: The structure stained in red with a lumen is the bladder.

Lower power lens: From the inner to the outer, the wall of the bladder can be divided into three layers: Mucosa, muscularis and adventitia. The mucous protrudes into cavity to form a plica, which is composed of the epithelium (transitional epithelium) and lamina propria. The superficial cells are large round or rectangular cells named as cap cells. The muscularis is thick and consisted of smooth muscle cells arranging into three layers that is difficult to distinguish. The adventitia is serosa.

Higher power lens: Observe the epithelium of the bladder.

(3) Observation key points: Three layers of the organ and epithelium of the mucosa.

III. Questions

1. Describe the structure and its relationship with the functions of the nephron.

2. Describe the structure and its relationship with the functions of the renal corpuscle.

3. Tell the differences between the proximal convoluted tubule and the distal convoluted tubule under the light microscope.

(Wu Xiaojing, Huang Shaoping)

第十五章
内分泌系统

一、实验目的

1. 掌握内分泌器官的共同特征；掌握肾上腺和垂体远侧部、神经部的光镜结构特点，并能加以区别。

2. 熟悉甲状腺的光镜结构；熟悉垂体中间部的光镜结构。

二、实验内容

1. 甲状腺（Thyroid gland）（彩图 76）

(1) 取材和染色：甲状腺，HE 染色。

(2) 观察：

肉眼：甲状腺组织块呈红色，其边缘的小块蓝色区为甲状旁腺。

低倍：甲状腺表面被覆一薄层结缔组织被膜。实质中有大小不等的球形甲状腺滤泡，并可见部分上皮细胞团，为没切到腔的滤泡。滤泡间为富含血管的结缔组织。

高倍：甲状腺滤泡上皮为单层立方上皮，细胞核圆，居细胞中央，腔中充满嗜酸性的胶质，被染成红色。在滤泡上皮或滤泡之间，可见滤泡旁细胞，体积大而圆，核圆，胞质浅染、清亮。

(3) 观察要点：滤泡及滤泡上皮细胞，滤泡旁细胞。

2. 肾上腺（Adrenal gland）（彩图 77～78）

(1) 取材和染色：肾上腺，HE 染色。

(2) 观察：

肉眼：最外侧为薄层结缔组织被膜，实质周围染色较深的为皮质，中间浅染部分为髓质。

低倍：被膜下的皮质依次分球状带、束状带和网状带。球状带染色较深，束状带最厚、染色浅淡；最内侧为网状带，染色较红。中央是髓质，染色较浅。

高倍:球状带细胞排列成团或球形,细胞小,染色深。束状带细胞平行排列成索,因富含脂滴被溶解,故染色较浅。网状带细胞排列成短索状并吻合成网,染色也较深。在皮质细胞索、团之间有丰富血窦。髓质中为髓质细胞(嗜铬细胞),胞体为较大的多边形,团、索状排列,其间有血窦和小静脉。

(3) 观察要点:区分皮、髓质,皮质的三条带;观察各种腺细胞的结构。

3. 垂体 (Hypophysis)(彩图 79~80)

(1) 取材和染色:垂体,HE 染色。

(2) 观察:

肉眼:标本染色较深的部分为腺垂体,主要是远侧部。染色较浅的部分为神经垂体,主要是神经部。

低倍:区分并观察远侧部和神经部的结构。远侧部染色深,大量腺细胞排列成团、成索状,其间的结缔组织富含血窦。神经部可见许多神经纤维和染成紫蓝色的神经胶质细胞核,胶质细胞胞质染色浅淡,不易区分,神经部也富含血窦。远侧部和神经部之间的狭小区域为中间部,内有许多大小不一的滤泡。

高倍:观察远侧部三种腺细胞。嗜酸性细胞体积较大,界限清楚,含大量红色嗜酸性颗粒。嗜碱性细胞体积也较大,界限清楚,含大量蓝色嗜碱性颗粒。嫌色细胞最多,较小,胞质不着色,界限不清,故可见成群的圆形细胞核。神经部内可见无髓神经纤维排列成束,神经胶质细胞又称垂体细胞,散在分布,垂体细胞较大,其胞质染色浅淡未能显示,故仅见细胞核。赫林体为大小不等、散在分布的均质状结构,嗜酸性,染成红色。

(3) 观察要点:远侧部、神经部和中间部,三种腺细胞、血窦。

三、思考题

1. 内分泌腺有何共同结构特征?
2. 试述甲状腺、肾上腺、脑垂体在光镜下的组织结构。
3. 垂体神经部在结构和功能上与下丘脑有何关系?

(黄少萍,朱丽娟)

Chapter 15
Endocrine System

Ⅰ. Experiment purpose

1. Master the general structures of organs of the endocrine system. Master the structures of the thyroid gland, adrenal gland, pars distalis, pars nervosa of the hypophysis under the light microscope.

2. Familiarity with the characters of the parafollicular cell and the pars intermedia under the light microscope.

Ⅱ. Experiment contents

1. Thyroid gland (Fig. 76)

(1) Materials: Thyroid gland, HE staining.

(2) Observe:

By eyes: The thyroid gland is red tissue and the little blue spot near the thyroid gland is the parathyroid.

Lower power lens: A thin connective tissue membrane cover the gland. In the parenchyma, there are many round follicles and between the follicles there are vessels, connective tissue and some cells clusters (maybe they are the glandular cells of the follicles)

Higher power lens: The wall of the follicles is consists of simple cuboidal epithelium with round nuclear in the center. There is red colloid in the lumen. The parafollicular cells, locates between the follicles or between the follicular cells, they are large with round nuclear and pale-staining cytoplasm.

(3) Observation key points: Follicles and follicular cells.

2. Adrenal gland (Figs. 77-78)

(1) Materials: Adrenal gland, HE staining.

(2) Observe:

By eyes: The organ is covered by the capsule. In the parenchyma, the dark part is the cortex and light part is the medulla.

Lower power lens: The cortex under the capsule can be divided into three layers, from the outer to the inner, they are zona glomerulosa, zona fasciculata and zona reticularis. Zona glomerulosa is dark stained, zona fasciculata is a light and thick one. The center of the gland is medulla.

Higher power lens: The cells of the cortex is irregular and their arrangement is also different. In the zona glomerulosa, the darker cells is arranged in round structure. In the zona fasciculata, the cells is arranged in cords and is in lighter stained because of containing numerous lipid droplets. In the zona reticularis, the cell coeds connect to each other forming a network in dark stain. Between the cells or cell cords there are many capillaries. In the medulla, the medullary cells are larger and polygonal, and arranged in clusters and cords, between them there are many capillaries too.

(3) Observation key points: cortex and medulla, zona glomerulosa, zona fasciculata and zona reticularis.

3. Hypophysis (Figs. 79-80)

(1) Materials: Hypophysis; HE stain.

(2) Observe:

By eyes: The tissue in dark stained is the adenohypophysis, most of them is the pars distalis. The lighter part is neurohypophysis, most of it is the pars nervosa.

Lower power lens: Observe the pars distalis and the pars nervosa carefully. First distinguish the pars distalis from pars nervosa. In pars distalis, the glandular cells are arranged in clusters or cords and connect to each other, between the cords there are many capillaries. In the pars nervosa, there are many nerve fibers, numerous blue nucleus of the glial cells and sinusoids. Between the pars distalis and the pars nervosa, is the pars intermedia containing many follicles.

Higher power lens: Observe the three kinds of glandular cells in the pars distalis carefully. The acidophils are larger cells with numerous red acidophilic granules in the cytoplasm and clear cell border. The basophiles are larger cells containing numerous blue basophilic granules and clear cell border too. There are more chromophobes than the other two kinds of cells, the chromophobes are lighter stained, the cell border is not clearly and you can only see the nucleus clearly. In the pars nervosa, there are nerve fibers arranged in bundles and nucleus of the glial cells (cytoplasm is stained so light that you can see clearly). The Herring bodies are different in shape and red homogenous structures.

(3) Observation key points: adenohypophysis, neurohypophysis, pars intermedia, three kinds of the endocrine cells.

III. Questions

1. What are the general structures of the organs of the endocrine system?

2. Describe the structures of the thyroid gland, adrenal gland, hypophysis under the light microscope.

3. Tell the relationship between the pars distalis and the pars nervosa.

(Huang Shaoping, Zhu Lijuan)

第十六章
男性生殖系统

一、实验目的

1. 掌握生精小管在光镜下的结构特点。掌握各级生精细胞和支持细胞的光镜结构特点。

2. 掌握间质细胞的结构,功能和分布。

3. 了解附睾输出小管和附睾管的结构特点。

二、实验内容

1. 睾丸（Testis）（彩图 81～82）

(1) 取材和染色:睾丸,HE 染色。

(2) 观察:

肉眼:为圆形的睾丸横切面。

低倍:可见生精小管的不同断面,管壁上皮为特殊的复层上皮。小管间的结缔组织为睾丸间质,含间质细胞。

高倍:① 生精小管:从基膜到腔面可见各级生精细胞排列有序,支持细胞位于其间,基底面附着在基膜上。

ⅰ 精原细胞:细胞体积较小,紧贴基膜,细胞核圆形,染色较深,偶见有丝分裂相。

ⅱ 初级精母细胞:位于精原细胞内侧,体积最大,由于多处于分裂前期,故核呈丝球状。

ⅲ 次级精母细胞:在初级精母细胞的内侧,形态与初级精母细胞相似,体积较小。由于其存在时间较短,故切片上不易找到。

ⅳ 精子细胞:位于精母细胞内侧,接近管腔面。体积较次级精母细胞更小,有些精子细胞渐变态形成精子,故呈长形或椭圆形,核延长,染色质致密故染色深。

ⅴ 精子:最靠近管腔或位于管腔内,呈蝌蚪状,头部埋于支持细胞的顶部胞质中,尾部朝向管腔。

ⅵ 支持细胞：细胞境界不清，基底面附着在基膜上，核浅染，呈三角形或不规则状，多位于精原细胞或精母细胞之间，胞质染色淡，顶部胞质可见埋于其中的精子头部。

② 间质细胞：生精小管间的疏松结缔组织为间质。可见间质细胞成群分布，细胞较大，呈椭圆形或多边形，胞核呈圆形，胞质嗜酸性。

(3) 观察要点：生精小管及各级生精细胞、支持细胞、间质细胞。

2. 附睾（Epididymis）（彩图 83～84）

(1) 取材和染色：附睾，HE 染色。

(2) 观察：

肉眼：组织分两部分，较大的为睾丸，另一部分为附睾，附于睾丸一侧，呈弧形。

低倍：可见两种不同的管腔断面：一种管壁较薄，上皮细胞高低不等，管腔面呈波浪状，为输出小管；另一种管壁较厚，管腔规则，为附睾管。

高倍：

① 输出小管：上皮为假复层柱状上皮，有纤毛的高柱状细胞和无纤毛的低柱状细胞相间排列，故腔面呈波浪状。基膜明显，其外有薄层平滑肌呈环形包绕。

② 附睾管：腔面整齐，上皮为假复层纤毛柱状上皮，游离面有静纤毛，腔内常有精子和分泌物。基膜外有一层平滑肌。

(3) 观察要点：区分输出小管和附睾管，观察上皮形态。

三、思考题

1. 试述光镜下各级生精细胞的结构。
2. 支持细胞的光镜结构特点是什么？你在光镜下能否观察清楚？
3. 睾丸间质细胞的有何光镜结构特点？有何功能？

（黄少萍，沈杨）

Chapter 16
Male Reproductive System

Ⅰ. Experiment purpose

1. Master the light microscope structure of seminiferous tubule. Master the characters of different kinds of spermatogenic cells and sertoli cells under the light microscope.

2. Master the structure, functions, and location of the interstitial cells (Leydig cells).

3. Understand the characters of the epididymis and the ductus deferens under the light microscope.

Ⅱ. Experiment contents

1. Testis (Figs. 81-82)

(1) Materials: Testis, HE staining.

(2) Observe:

By eyes: The tissue includes two organs: The larger round-shaped organ is testis. Other one is the section of epididymis.

Lower power lens: A lot of cross section with different shaped of seminiferous tubules can be seen in the parenchyma. The seminiferous tubule is mainly lined by seminiferous epithelium, consisting of Sertoli cells and 5-8 layers of spermatogenic cells. Between the tubules is the interstitial tissue (connective tissue), containing interstitial cells.

Higher power lens:

① Seminiferous tubules: From the basal part to the apical surface of the tubule, different kinds of spermatogenic cells can be seen in order. The Sertoli cells are also located in the wall of the tubule. It is difficult to figure out the Sertoli cells.

ⅰ Spermatogenic cells: Spermatogonia base on the basement of the tubules. They are relatively small round cells with oval-shaped nucleus containing fine and dense chromatins. ⅱ Primary spermatocytes are the largest cells lie on the spermatogonia. They always have a large, flocculus-like nucleus. ⅲ Secondary spermatocytes are smaller than the spermatocytes. Because they not need to duplicate the chromatins and quickly enter the next cell division, so seldom can be seen in the sections. ⅳ Spermatids are small round cells with deeply stained nuclei, situating adjacent to the lumen. ⅴ Spermatozoa like a tadpole, consists of two part namely head and tail. Their head always embed in the apical cytoplasm of the sertoli cells with tails extending to the lumen. ⅵ Sertoli cells: The outline of Sertoli cell is not obvious. They base on the basement and the cytoplasm extending to the lumen. Their nuclei are large ovoid or triangular in shape, pale-stained, and nucleoli are often prominent. The cytoplasm of cells are acidophilic.

② Leydig cells: They are located in interstitial tissue in groups. The cells are large, round or polygonal and acidophilic cells with a large, round and pale-stained nucleus.

(3) Observation key points: Seminiferous tubules, structures of different kinds of spermatogenic cells and the Sertoli cells, location and characters of the Leydig cells.

2. Epididymis (Figs. 83-84)

(1) Materials: Epididymis, HE staining.

(2) Observe:

By eyes: The tissue includes two organs: the larger organ is testis, the other one is the section of epididymis attaching to one side of testis, and is curved.

Lower power lens: In the epididymis, two different ducts can be seen. One kind of ducts has wavy lumen surface, and a thin wall containing high and low epithelial cells, these ducts are efferent ductules. The other has a larger lumen, thicker wall and regular lumen. These ducts are epididymal ducts.

Higher power lens: ① Efferent duct: the epithelium is stratified columnar epithelium, consisting of high columnar cells with no cilli and low columnar cells. The basement is clear and is surrounded by thin layer of smooth muscle.

② The epididymal duct has a larger lumen and thick wall, which is consisting of high pseudostratified columnar cells with long stereocilia. Outside the basement membrane, there is a thin layer of smooth muscle cells. In the lumen, spermatozoa and acidophilic secretion always can be seen.

(3) Observation key points: Efferent ductules, epididymal ducts and high pseudostratified columnar cells, basement membrane.

III. Questions

1. Describe the structure of seminiferous tubule and different types of spermatogenic cells of spermatogenesis.

2. What are the structure and function of the sertoli cell? Can you observe the outline of the Sertoli cells clearly in our section?

3. What are the structural characters and function of the Leydig cells?

(Huang Shaoping, Shen Yang)

第十七章
女性生殖系统

一、实验目的

1. 掌握卵巢的组织结构，掌握各级卵泡的结构特点。
2. 掌握子宫和黄体的组织结构。
3. 熟悉输卵管的组织结构。

二、实验内容

1. 卵巢(Ovary)(彩图 85～86)

(1) 取材和染色：卵巢，HE 染色。

(2) 观察：

肉眼：可见椭圆形组织，外周紫蓝色的部分为皮质，中央红色的一小部分为髓质。

低倍：卵巢表面被覆单层扁平或立方细胞，上皮下方为薄层的致密结缔组织白膜，细胞多，纤维少。外周部分为皮质，可见各级卵泡、闭锁卵泡、黄体及致密的结缔组织基质。切片中未见成熟卵泡。中央部分为髓质，由疏松结缔组织组成，富含血管和神经纤维。较多结缔组织和血管进出的一侧为卵巢门部。

高倍：选择典型的卵泡和黄体详细观察。

① 各级卵泡：

ⅰ 原始卵泡：位于皮质浅层，数量多，体积小。由中央的初级卵母细胞和周围一层扁平的卵泡细胞构成。卵母细胞核大而圆，浅染，空泡状，核仁清楚。

ⅱ 初级卵泡：体积较原始卵泡大，由中央一个较大的初级卵母细胞和周围单层立方或多层卵泡细胞组成。初级卵母细胞和周围卵泡间出现一层嗜酸性膜，均质状，称透明带。

ⅲ 次级卵泡：体积更大，卵泡细胞增至 6～12 层。卵泡细胞间出现卵泡腔，其中有卵泡液。卵母细胞及周围的卵泡细胞向卵泡腔突起呈丘状，称卵丘。卵泡腔周围的卵泡细胞称颗粒层，透明带周围的一层卵泡细胞呈放射状排列，为放射冠。卵泡外面的结缔组织形成卵泡膜,其内层细胞多,血管丰富,外层纤维多。

ⅳ 成熟卵泡:未见成熟卵泡。

ⅴ 闭锁卵泡:卵母细胞退化,透明带皱缩,卵泡细胞溶解。部分卵泡膜细胞可分化为间质腺,细胞肥大,多边形,胞质嗜酸性并充满脂滴,常被结缔组织分隔成团、索状。

② 黄体:为染色浅淡的细胞团,体积很大,其中富含毛细血管。黄体细胞分两种。ⅰ 粒黄体细胞,胞体较大,胞质内充满脂滴,着色浅,呈空泡状;ⅱ 膜黄体细胞,胞体较小,胞质着色较深。

③ 基质:为结缔组织,含有大量的梭形细胞,含有退化的闭锁卵泡。

(3) 观察要点:区分皮质和髓质,观察各级卵泡、闭锁卵泡和黄体的结构。

2. 子宫(Uterus)

(1) 取材和染色:子宫体,HE 染色。

(2) 观察:

肉眼:染成淡紫色的结构为子宫内膜,深红色较厚的部分为肌层。

低倍:依次观察子宫壁的三层结构。

① 子宫内膜:由单层柱状上皮和固有层(结缔组织)构成。内膜浅层较厚的部分称为功能层。下方为基底层,较薄,近肌层且着色较深(红色)。功能层和基底层交界处,有许多螺旋动脉,多为其横切面。固有层可见大量子宫腺。

② 肌层:很厚,分层不明显,为成束排列的平滑肌,其间富含血管。

③ 外膜:为薄层的结缔组织和一层间皮。

高倍:重点观察分泌期子宫内膜。

① 上皮:单层柱状,由少量纤毛细胞和大量无纤毛的分泌细胞组成。

② 固有层:为结缔组织,细胞多、纤维少,基质细胞肥大,呈圆形或多边形,核大,浅染,胞质着色浅,称前蜕膜细胞。

③ 子宫腺:为单层柱状形成的管状腺,腺体弯曲,腺腔大而不规则,内有许多分泌物。

注意观察子宫内膜的厚度、腺体的形态及内含物变化、螺旋动脉高度、基质细胞形态、基质水肿程度等,判断子宫内膜处于月经周期中的哪一期。

(3) 观察要点:区分子宫内膜分层各层,观察子宫内膜厚度,观察子宫腺、螺旋动脉、基质细胞等结构。

3. 输卵管(Oviduct)

(1) 取材和染色:输卵管壶腹部,HE 染色。

(2) 观察:

肉眼:为管腔不明显的圆形结构,近腔部分染成紫色的是黏膜,周围是肌层和浆膜,染成红色。

低倍:由内向外管壁分黏膜、肌层和浆膜三层。

① 黏膜:管腔形态不规则,黏膜由单层柱状上皮和固有层组成,向管腔突出形成许多有分支的纵形皱襞。

② 肌层:较薄,分内环、外纵两层平滑肌,分界不清。

③ 浆膜:为富含血管的疏松结缔组织和一层间皮构成。

高倍:观察黏膜结构。

① 上皮:单层柱状上皮,为大量的纤毛细胞和少量分泌细胞构成。

② 固有层:疏松结缔组织,富含血管及少量散在平滑肌。

(3) 观察要点:输卵管的三层结构、黏膜上皮和黏膜皱襞。

三、思考题

1. 原始卵泡、初级卵泡和次级卵泡在结构上有何不同?

2. 什么是黄体?它由哪两类细胞组成?各自产生什么激素?

3. 月经周期分哪几期?子宫内膜发生哪些变化?这些变化受卵巢哪些激素的调节?

(沈杨,黄少萍)

Chapter 17
Female Reproductive System

Ⅰ. Experiment purpose

1. Master the structure of the ovary, the features of the follicles in different developing stages.

2. Master the structures of the uterus and the structures of corpus luteum.

3. Be familiar with the structures of the oviduct.

Ⅱ. Experiment contents

1. Ovary (Figs. 85-86)

(1) Materials: Ovary, HE staining.

(2) Observe:

By eyes: The outer part of the ovary with some big or small vacuoles is the cortex, and the inner small part is the medulla.

Lower power lens: The ovary is covered with simple cuboidal or simple squamous epithelium (germinal epithelium). Beneath the epithelium is the albuginea, the outer part of the parenchyma is cortex, which contains ovarian follicles of various developing stages and corpus luteum, the narrow central region is the medulla composed of loose connective tissue.

Higher power lens:

① Ovarian follicles: ⅰ Primordial follicle: The follicles are small in size, and the most in number. They locate in the periphery of the cortex and accumulate in groups. There is a primary oocyte in the middle of the follicle. A layer flattened follicular cells surrounding the oocyte is simple epithelium. ⅱ Primary follicle: It consists of a primary oocyte and a layer of cuboidal or more layers follicular cells enveloping the primary oocyte. An thick acidophilic membrane is situated between the oocyte and follicular cells, it is zona pellucida. ⅲ Secondary follicle: The secondary follicle is vesicle-shaped and contains a follicular antrum. The wall of the follicles is composed of stratified follicular cells, named granular layer. The oocyte and its surrounding radial granular cell (corona radiata) protrudes toward the antrum form the cumulus oophorus. The connective tissue around the follicle forms the theca folliculi. There are no visible boundary between the theca folliculi and surrounding connective tissue. ⅳ Mature follicle: It is not easy to be seen, so it is not necessary to observe. ⅴ Atretic follicle: The oocyte degenerates, zona pellucida shrinks, follicle cell is lysed. Some theca cells may differentiate into stromal glands, the cells of gland are hypertrophic, polygonal, eosinophilic and filled with lipid droplets, and are often separated by connective tissue into clumps or cords.

② Corpus luteum: In the cortex, some larger corpus luteum can be seen. The corpus luteum contains two kinds of lutein cells: The lutein cells are the granular lutein cells, they are bigger, polygonal cells with vacuolated cytoplasm. The theca lutein cells are smaller and stain more strongly, and they are less in number, located in the folds of the wall of the corpus luteum.

③ Interstitial tissue: It is the connective tissue. atresic follicles are characterized by atrophy and disappearance of both the oocyte and the follicular cells.

(3) Observation key points: To distinguish the cortex and medulla, different kinds of the follicles, corpus luteum, and so on.

2. Uterus

(1) Materials: Uterus, HE staining.

(2) Observe:

By eyes: The layer stained in purple is the endometrium, the thick red layer is the myometrium.

Lower power lens:

① Endometrium: It is consisted of a simple columnar epithelium and lamina propria (connective tissue). The thick superficial layer of the endometrium is the functional layer, and the lower part is the basal layer. Between the functional layer and the basal layer, there are many cross-section of the spiral arteries. Also, numerous uterine glands can be seen in the lamina propria.

② Myometrium: It is consisted of smooth muscle cell, they are arranged in three layers and it is not easy to distinguish their boundaries.

③ Perimetrium: It is composed of a thin layer of connective tissue covered with mesothelium.

Higher power lens：

① Epithelium：The simple columnar epithelium is composed of a small number of ciliated cells and a large number of non-ciliated secretory cells.

② Lamina propria：It is connective tissue with more cells and less fibers，the stromal cells are hypertrophic，round or polygonal，with pale stained nuclei and cytoplasm，called predecidual cells.

③ Uterine glands：They are the single columnar tubular gland with curved glands and large irregular glandular cavities with many secretions.

Observe the thickness of the endometrium，glandular morphology and its secretion，height of the spiral artery，morphology of stromal cell，edema of the endometrium. Can you determine which stages of the menstrual cycle of the endometrium is in your section?

(3) Observation key points：Three layers of the uterus：endometrium，myometrium，perimetrium，the functional layer and the basal layer，predecidual cells，uterine glands，spiral artery，and so on.

3. Oviduct

(1) Materials：Oviduct，HE staining.

(2) Observe：

By eyes：Lumen of the oviduct is not obvious，the purple part near the lumen is mucosa，surrounded by muscle layer stained in red and serosa.

Lower power lens：From the inner to the outer，the wall of the oviduct can be divided into 3 layers：mucosa，muscularis，serosa.

① Mucosa：It is consisted of a simple columnar epithelium and lamina propria. The mucosa protrudes into the lumen to form many branching longitudinal plica mucosa resulting in an irregular lumen.

② Muscularis：It is a thin layer consisting of smooth muscle cell，it can be divided into inner circular and outer longitudinal layers with not clear boundary.

③ Serosa：It is consisted of connective tissue rich in blood vessel and mesothelium (a simple squamous epithelium).

Higher power lens：

① Epithelium：It is simple columnar epithelium which is composed of a large number of ciliated cells and a small number of non-ciliated secretory cells.

② Lamina propria：It is loose connective tissue rich in blood vessels and few cells.

(3) Observation key points：Three layers of the oviduct，epithelium and the plica mocusa.

III. Questions

1. What are differences in the structure among the primordial follicles, primary follicles and secondary follicles?

2. What is corpus luteum? Tell the structure and function of the corpus luteum.

3. How many stages are included in the menstrual cycle? What changes does the endometrium taken place in each stage of the menstrual cycle? Which ovarian hormones regulate these changes in the endometrium?

(Shen Yang, Huang Shaoping)

第十八章
胚胎学总论一

一、实验目的

1. 掌握两性生殖细胞的成熟以及精子的获能。
2. 掌握受精的部位及过程，卵裂、胚泡的结构及形成过程。
3. 掌握内细胞群的分化，二胚层胚盘的结构及形成过程。
4. 掌握三胚层胚盘的形成过程及其早期分化。

二、实验内容

1. 卵裂和胚泡(Cleavage and blastocyst)(彩图 87～89)

(1) 标本：卵裂模型、胚泡模型。

(2) 观察：

① 卵裂：观察二细胞、四细胞、八细胞期的模型。受精卵在透明带进行卵裂，卵裂球(子细胞)的数目逐渐增多，体积逐渐变小。

② 桑葚胚：观察桑葚胚模型。卵裂球数目达 12～16 个时，形成外观如桑葚的细胞团，称桑葚胚。可见卵裂球体积较八细胞期更小。

③ 胚泡：观察胚泡模型。卵裂球数目达 100 个左右，胚如囊泡状，称胚泡。胚泡的壁由单层细胞组成，胚泡中央有胚泡腔，腔内一侧的细胞团为内细胞群。内细胞群一侧的滋养层细胞称极滋养层。

(3) 观察要点：二细胞期、四细胞期、八细胞期、桑葚胚及胚泡的结构。

2. 二胚层胚盘分化(Differentiation of the bilaminar germ disc)(彩图 90)

(1) 标本：内细胞群模型。

(2) 观察：

① 内细胞群：观察内细胞群的分化模型。可见内细胞群增殖，逐渐形成两层细胞，近胚泡腔的一层立方形细胞，称下胚层；其上方的一层柱状细胞，称上胚层。上下胚层形成

二胚层胚盘。随后，上下胚层的细胞增殖，上胚层上方出现羊膜腔，下胚层下方出现卵黄囊。

② 滋养层：滋养层细胞迅速增殖并形成两层：内层细胞界限清楚，为细胞滋养层；外层细胞多，融合成较厚的一层，为合体滋养层。

③ 胚外中胚层：胚泡腔出现星形松散的细胞及基质，称胚外中胚层。随后，胚外中胚层中出现一个大的腔，称胚外体腔。胚外体腔将胚外中胚层分为两层：胚外体壁中胚层覆盖在卵黄囊的表面；胚外脏壁中胚层覆盖细胞滋养层的内表面。

(3) 观察要点：内细胞群、滋养层及胚外中胚层等结构。

3. 三胚层胚盘分化(Differentiation of the trilaminar germ disc)(彩图 91～92)

(1) 标本：三胚层胚盘、胚体卷折模型、神经管分化模型。

(2) 观察：

① 三胚层胚盘：上胚层细胞增殖快，在胚盘尾端中线上形成一条细胞索，称原条；原条的上胚层细胞进入并置换了下胚层细胞，下胚层改称为内胚层；并在上胚层和内胚层之间扩展形成新的一层，为中胚层；至此，原来的上胚层改称为外胚层。内、中、外三个胚层形成三胚层胚盘。

② 外胚层分化：盘状的胚胎卷折形成类似圆柱状的结构。外胚层中线部分细胞增殖形成神经外胚层：神经板→神经沟→神经管，最后神经管的前神经孔和后神经孔闭合，神经管分化为脑、脊髓。其余的外胚层包裹胚体，分化形成皮肤的表皮。

③ 中胚层分化：脊索两侧的中胚层由内向外依次分为下列三部分：

ⅰ 轴旁中胚层：由上而下断裂形成体节，左右对称，共 42～44 对。

ⅱ 间介中胚层：介于轴旁中胚层和侧中胚层之间

ⅲ 侧中胚层：出现胚内体腔，故侧中胚层被分为体壁中胚层和脏壁中胚层两部分。

④ 内胚层分化：内胚层卷褶形成头尾走向的管道，为原始消化管，位于胚胎中央。

(3) 观察要点：卵裂球的结构，二胚层胚盘结构，三胚层胚盘的形成、结构及分化。

三、思考题

1. 什么是卵裂？胚泡包括哪几个部分？

2. 什么是二胚层胚盘？什么是三胚层胚盘？

3. 试述三胚层胚盘各分化为哪些结构。

(卢莹，黄少萍)

Chapter 18
General embryology Ⅰ

Ⅰ. Experiment purpose

1. Master the maturation of the germ cells in male and female. Master the process of the capacitation of the sperm.

2. Master the site and process of the fertilization, the process and structure of the cleavage and the blastocyst.

3. Master the differentiation of the inner cell group, the structure and formation process of the bilaminar germ disc.

4. Master the formation process and early differentiation of the trilaminar germ disc.

Ⅱ. Experiment contents

1. Cleavage and blastocyst (Figs. 87-89)

(1) Materials: Models of cleavage and blastocyst.

(2) Observe:

① Cleavage: Observe the two-cell, four-cell, eight-cell model. Zygote go on mitosis cleavage in the space surrounded by the zona pellucida, the number of blastomeres (daughter cells) gradually increased, the volume of the blastomeres gradually decreased.

② Morula: When the number of blastomeres reached 12-16, the zygote looked like mulberries, is called morula. Note that the size of the blastomere is smaller than that of the eight-cell stage.

③ Blastocyst: When the number of blastomeres is about 100, and the embryo is like vesicle, it is called blastocyst. The wall of the blastocyst is composed of monolayer cells, named as trophoblast. There is a cavity in the center of the blastocyst, in one side of cavity, there is a mass of cells called inner cell mass. The trophoblast covering the inner cell mass is call polar trophoblast.

(3) Observation key points: Observe the cleavage in the two-cell stage, four-cell stage, eight-cell stage, and structure of morula and blastocyst.

2. Differentiation of the bilaminar germ disc (Fig. 90)

(1) Materials: Models of blastocyst inner cell mass.

(2) Observe:

① Inner cell mass: It can be seen that the inner cell group proliferate and gradually form two layers of cells: one layer of cubic cells near the blastocyst cavity, which is called the hypoblast. The upper layer of columnar cells is called the epiblast. The upper layer and the lower layer of the embryo form the bilaminar germ disc. Subsequently, cells in the upper and lower layers proliferates, on the epiblast, there is a amniotic cavity; under the hypoblast, there is a yolk sac.

② Trophoblast: Trophoblastic cells rapidly proliferate and form two layers: the inner layer cells with clear cell boundaries are called cytotrophoblast; Outer layer of cells, fuse into a thicker layer, for the syncytiotrophoblast.

③ Extraembryonic mesoderm: Loose star-shaped cells and matrix appear in the blastocyst cavity, which is called extraembryonic mesoderm. Subsequently, a large cavity appearing in the extraembryonic mesoderm is called the extraembryonic coelom. The coelom divides the extraembryonic mesoderm into two layers: the splanchnic mesoderm covers the outer surface of the yolk sac; the somatic mesoderm covers the inner surface of the cytotrophoblast.

(3) Observation key points: Inner cell mass, cytotrophoblast and the syncytiotrophoblast, extraembryonic mesoderm.

3. Differentiation of the trilaminar germ disc (Figs. 91-92)

(1) Materials: Model of trilaminar germ disc, model of embryo body folding and neural tube.

(2) Observe:

① Trilaminar germ disc: Epiblast cells proliferate rapidly and form a cell cord on the midline at the end of the embryo disc, which is called the primitive streak; The cell of primitive streak proliferates, enters and replaces the hypoblast cells which renamed as endoderm; also, a new layer is formed between the two layers, which is called mesoderm. Later, the original epiblast was renamed ectoderm. These three layers form the trilaminar germ disc.

② Differentiation of the ectoderm: The trilaminar germ disc folds into a cylindrical structure. Some cells in the midline of the ectoderm proliferate to form the neuroectoderm: neural plate→neural sulcus→neural tube. Finally, the anterior and posterior neural foramen of the neural tube are closed, and the neural tube differentiates into brain and spinal cord. The remaining ectoderm envelops the body of the embryo and differentiates into the epidermis of the skin.

③ Differentiation of the mesoderm: The mesoderm in both sides of the notochord is divided into the following three parts from the inside to the outside:

ⅰ Paraxial mesoderm: from the top to the bottom to form a segment, bilateral symmetry, a total of 42-44 pairs.

ⅱ Mesoderm: between the axial mesoderm and the lateral mesoderm

ⅲ Lateral mesoderm: the body cavity in the embryo appears, so it is divided into the body wall mesoderm and the visceral wall mesoderm.

④ Differentiation of the endoderm: Endoderm curls to form a tube from the top to tail, which is the original digestive tube and located in the center of the embryo.

(3) Observation key points: Observe the volume of blastomeres, the structure of bilaminar germ disc, the formation, structure and the differentiation of trilaminar germ disc.

Ⅲ. Questions

1. What is cleavage? How many parts does a blastocyst consist of?
2. What is bilaminar germ disc? What is the trilaminar germ disc?
3. Tell the differentiation of the trilaminar germ disc.

(Lu Ying, Huang Shaoping)

第十九章
胚胎学总论二

一、实验目的

1. 掌握胎膜的组成,绒毛膜的结构和功能,羊膜结构和功能。
2. 掌握卵黄囊、尿囊在胚胎发育中的意义,脐带的结构和意义。
3. 胎盘的结构、胎盘的血液循环与胎盘膜组成。

二、实验内容

1. 胎膜(Fetal membrane)(彩图 93~96)

(1) 标本:胎膜模型。

(2) 观察:

① 绒毛膜:绒毛膜板由滋养层和胚外体壁中胚层组成。绒毛膜板和其表面的绒毛组成绒毛膜,随后绒毛膜由于血供的不同,发育为两部分:平滑绒毛膜和丛密绒毛膜。绒毛干的发育经历三阶段:ⅰ初级绒毛干;中轴为细胞滋养层。ⅱ次级绒毛干;中轴为胚外中胚层。ⅲ三级绒毛干;中轴的胚外中胚层分化,出现结缔组织和血管。

② 羊膜:由羊膜上皮和胚外中胚层构成。

③ 卵黄囊:胚体卷褶以后,卵黄囊退化成卵黄管,最后形成缩窄形成卵黄蒂,被包裹在脐带中。

④ 尿囊:为细长的盲囊,也被包裹在脐带中。

⑤ 脐带:胚体卷褶,由羊膜包裹卵黄囊、尿囊、体蒂、脐血管等结构并缩窄形成的索状结构。

(3) 观察要点:绒毛膜及各级绒毛干;羊膜、卵黄囊、尿囊和脐带的结构。

2. 胎盘(Placenta)(彩图 96)

(1) 标本:妊娠子宫模型和胎盘模型。

(2) 观察:

① 丛密绒毛膜:可见绒毛膜发育为平滑绒毛膜和丛密绒毛膜。丛密绒毛膜长入母体子宫。丛密绒毛膜和母体的基蜕膜共同构成胎盘。

② 胎盘:圆盘状,中央厚周边薄。胎儿面有羊膜覆盖,光滑,近中央处有脐带附着;母体面粗糙,由基蜕膜构成的胎盘隔将其分隔成15～30个胎盘小叶。

③ 胎盘膜:由合体滋养层、细胞滋养层及基膜、薄层的绒毛结缔组织、毛细血管基膜和内皮组成。

(3) 观察要点:胎盘及胎盘膜的结构。

三、思考题

1. 什么是绒毛膜板? 什么是绒毛膜? 绒毛干发育分几个阶段?
2. 胎膜包括哪些部分? 各有什么功能或临床意义?
3. 胎盘由哪些部分组成? 胎盘膜的组成成分及功能是什么?

(李苏影,黄少萍)

Chapter 19
General embryology Ⅱ

Ⅰ. Experiment purpose

1. Master the composition of fetal membrane, the structure and function of chorionic membrane, and the structure and function of amniotic membrane.

2. Grasp the significance of yolk sac and allantoic sac in embryo development.

3. Master the structure of umbilical cord, placenta, master the blood circulation of placenta and components of the placenta membrane.

Ⅱ. Experiment contents

1. Fetal membrane (Figs. 93-96)

(1) Materials: Fetal membrane model.

(2) Observe:

① Chorionic membrane: The chorionic membrane plate consists of the trophoblast layer and the mesoderm of the ectoderm. The chorionic lamella and the villi on its surface make up the chorionic membrane, which then develops into smooth chorionic membrane and dense chorionic membrane. Stem villi: ⅰ Primary stem villi: the axis of the stem villi is the cell trophoblast layer. ⅱ Secondary stem villi: The axis of the secondary villi is the extraembryonic mesoderm. ⅲ Tertiary stem villi, the central axis of the villi is differentiated, containing connective tissue and blood vessels.

② Amniotic membrane: Composed of amniotic epithelium and ectoderm.

③ Yolk sac: After the embryo body is folded, the yolk sac degenerates into the yolk tube, and finally forms the yolk peduncle, which is wrapped in the umbilical cord.

④ Allantoic sac: A slender blind sac also encased in the umbilical cord.

⑤ Umbilical cord: The embryo body is rolled and pleated, which is a cord-like structure formed by the amnion wrapping and narrowing the yolk sac, allantoic sac, body pedicle and umbilical blood tube.

(3) Observation key points: Observe the chorionic plate, chorionic membrane and villi; The structure of amniotic membrane, yolk sac, allantoic sac, umbilical cord,

2. Placenta (Fig. 96)

(1) Materials: Pregnant uterus model and placenta model.

(2) Observe:

① Chorion frondosum: The chorion develops quickly, the part near the decidua capsularis degenerates and forms the chorion laeve; the other part of the chorion grows into the mother's uterus, the villi grows well and forms the chorion frondosum. The chorion frondosum and decidua basalis of the mother constitute the placenta.

② Placenta: It is disc-shaped, thick in the center and thin in the periphery. The surface facing to the fetus is covered with amniotic membrane, so it is smooth and attached by umbilical cord near the center. The surface facing to the decidua basalis is rough, and the placental septum composed of basal decidua divides it into 15～30 placental lobules.

③ Placental membrane: It is composed of syncytiotrophoblast, cytotrophoblast, basal membrane, thin layer of villous connective tissue, capillary basement membrane and endothelium.

(3) Observation key points: The structure of chorionic frondosum, placenta and placental membrane.

III. Questions

1. What is a chorionic plaque? What is chorionic membrane? How many grades of villi can be found during their developing process?

2. What are the components of the membranes? What are their functional or clinical implications?

3. What are the components of the placenta? What are the components and functions of placenta?

(Li Suying, Huang Shaoping)

彩色图谱

Figures of Histology and Embryology

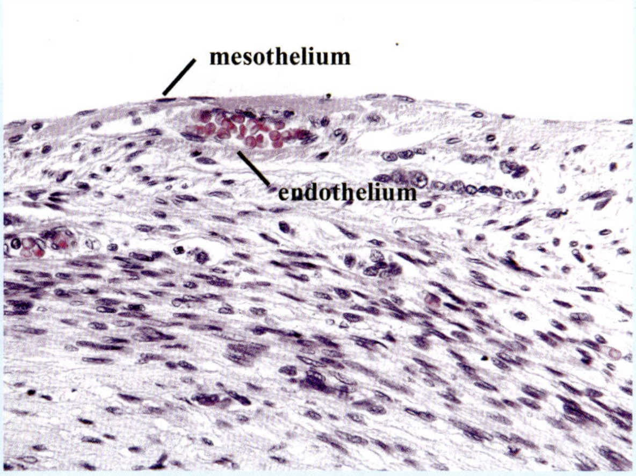

Fig. 1 Simple squamous epithelium (10×40)

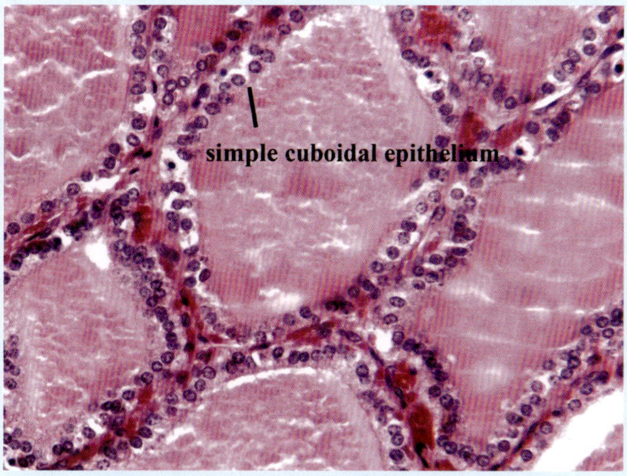

Fig. 2 Simple cuboidal epithelium (10×40)

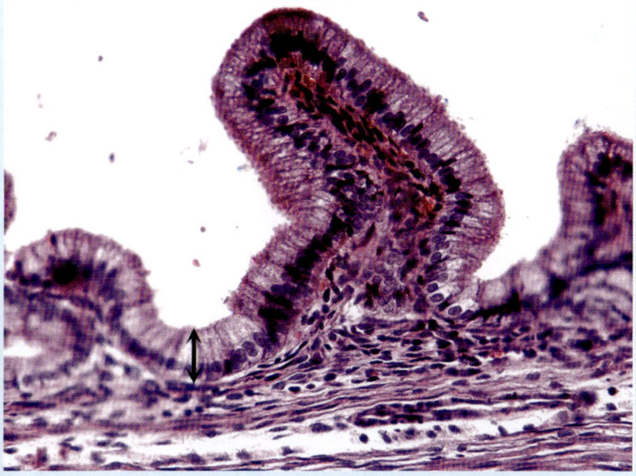

Fig. 3 Simple columnar epithelium
(10×40)

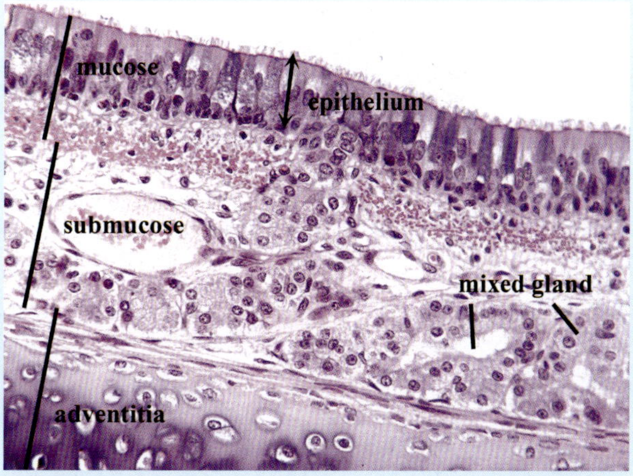

Fig. 4 Pseudostratified ciliated columnar epithelium
(10×40)

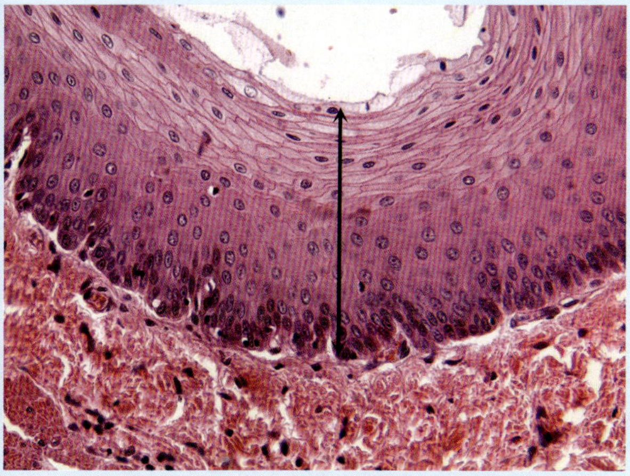

Figure 5 Stratified squmous epithelium
(10×40)

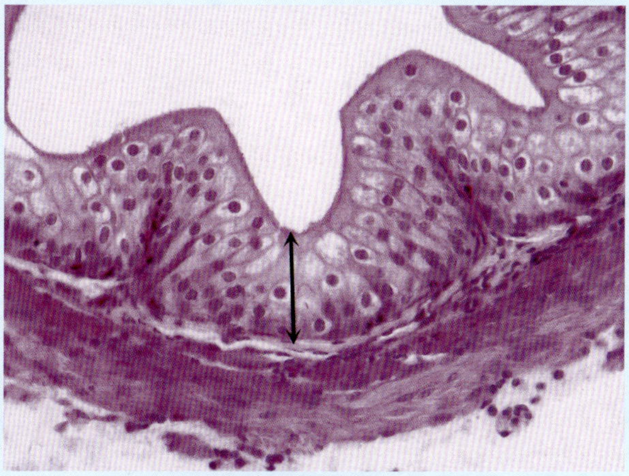

Fig. 6 Transitional epithelium
(10×40)

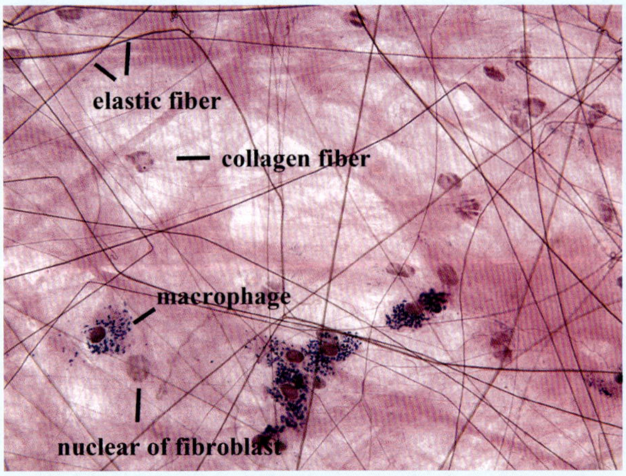

Fig. 7 Loose connective tissue stretched preparation (10×40)

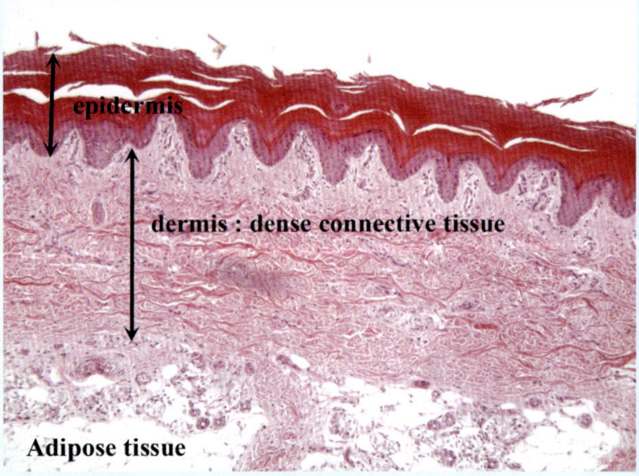

Fig. 8 Loose, dense connective tissue and adipose tissue (10×10)

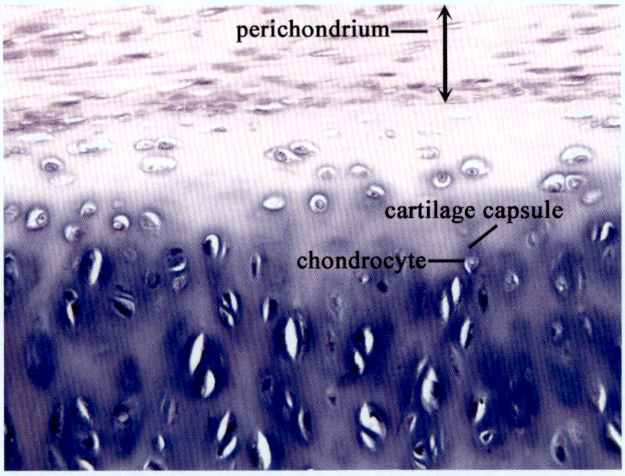

Fig. 9 Hyaline cartilage (10×10)

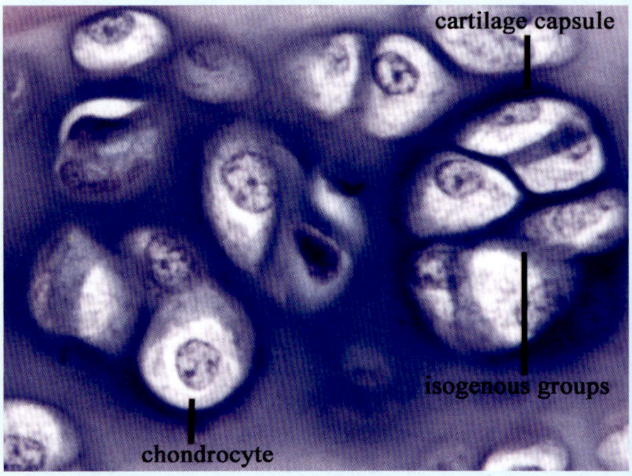

Fig. 10 Hyaline cartilage (10×40)

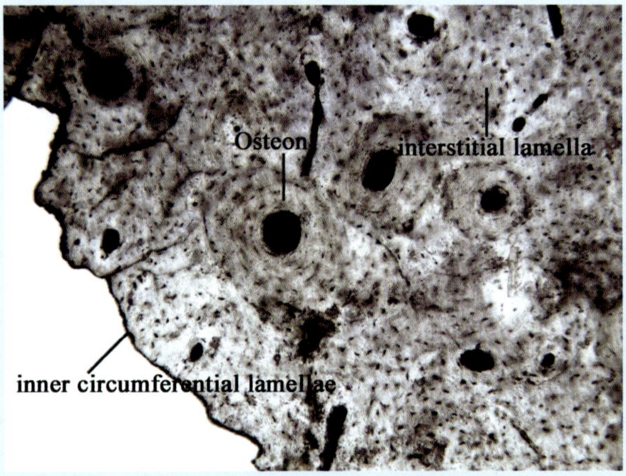

Fig. 11 Compact bone (10×10)

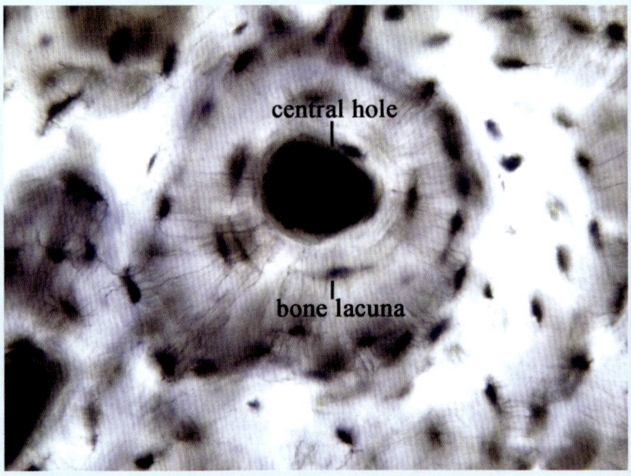

Fig. 12 Havers' system (10×40)

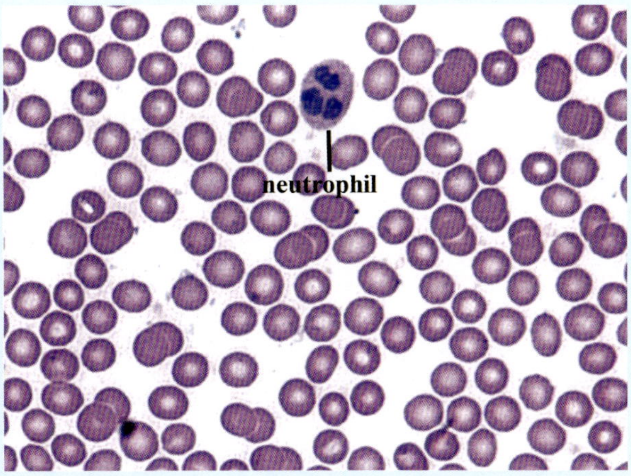

Fig. 13 Neutrophil (10×40)

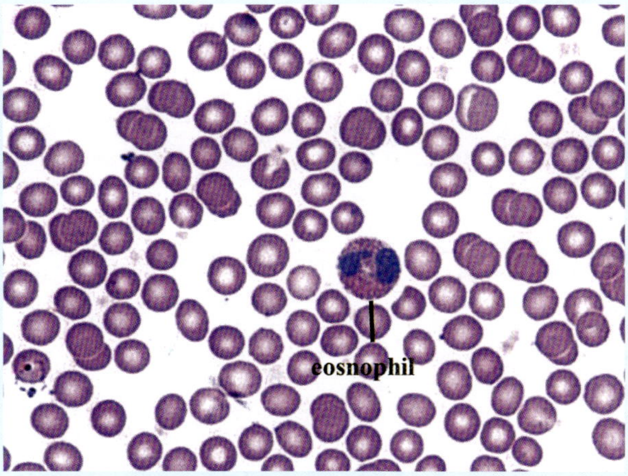

Fig. 14 Eosnophil (10×40)

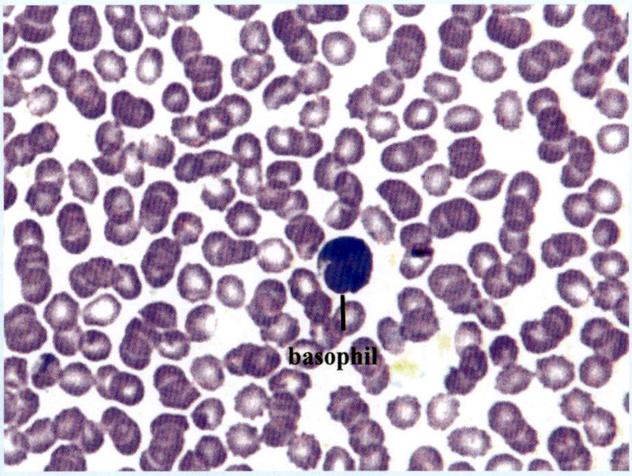

Fig. 15 Basophil (10×40)

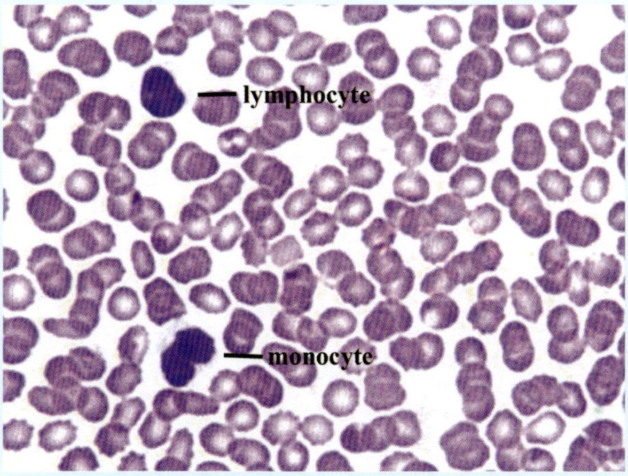

Fig. 16 Monocyte (10×40)

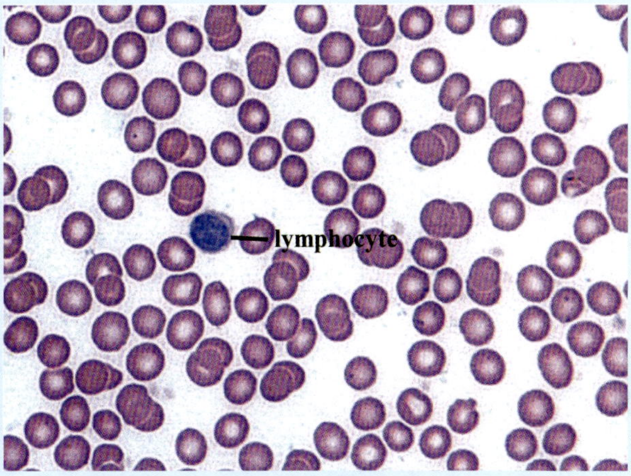

Fig. 17 Lymphocyte (10×40)

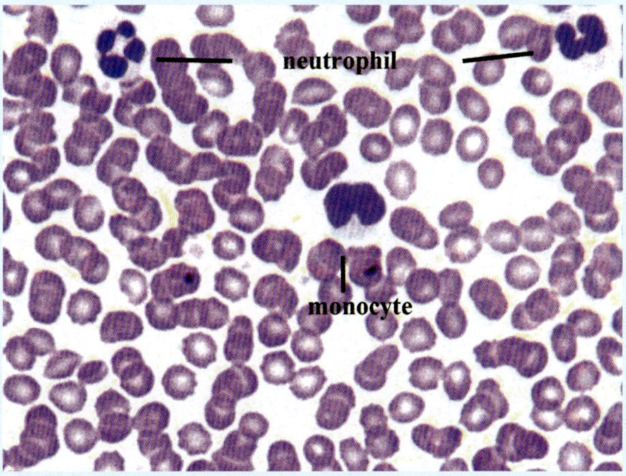

Fig. 18 Neutrophil+Monocyte (10×40)

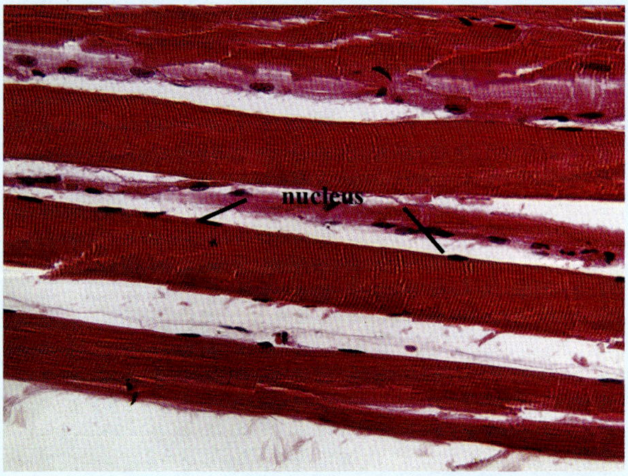

Fig. 19: Longitudinal section of skeletal muscle (10×40)

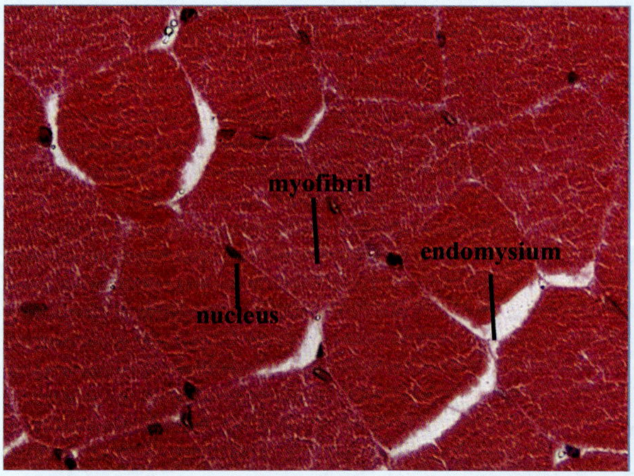

Fig. 20 Transverse section of skeletal muscle (10×40)

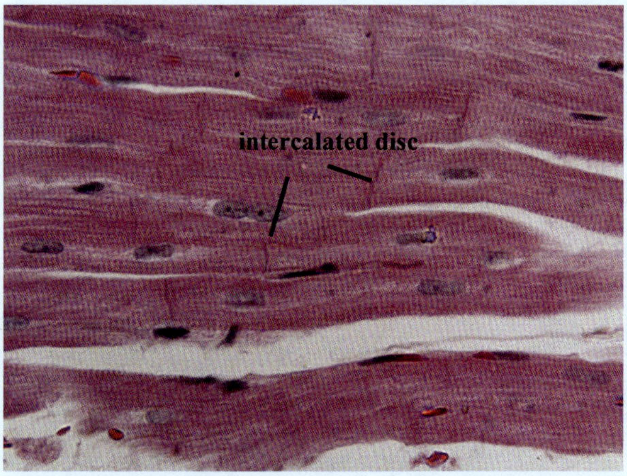

Fig. 21 Longitudinal section of cardiac muscle (10×40)

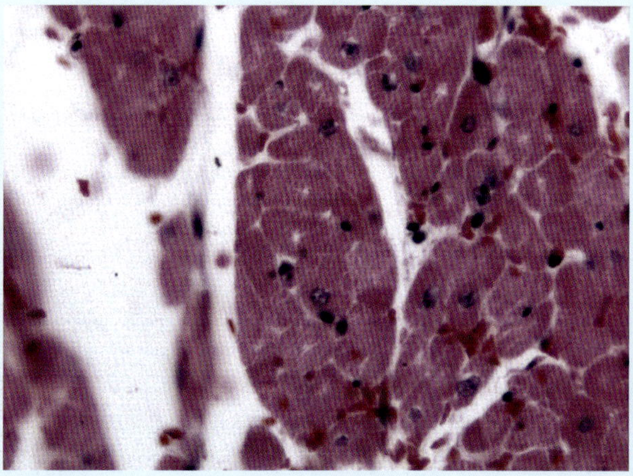

Fig. 22 Transverse section of cardiac muscle (10×40)

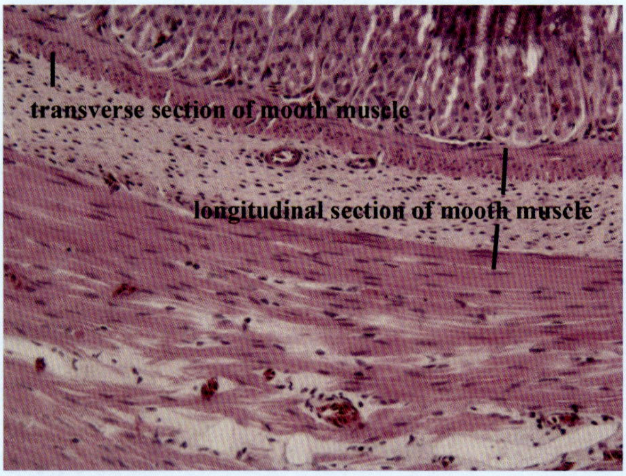

Fig. 23 Smooth muscle (10×10)

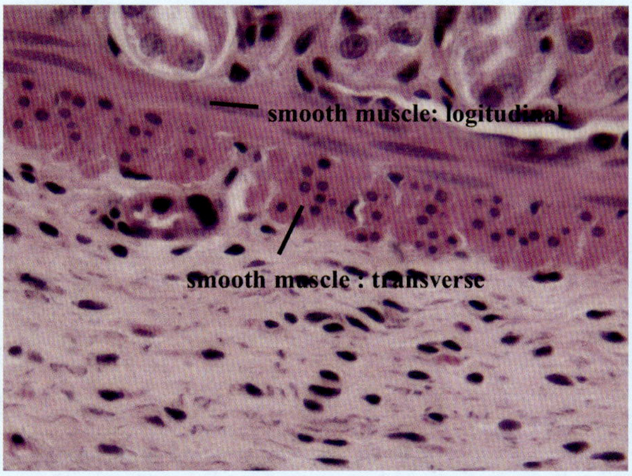

Fig. 24 Smooth muscle (10×40)

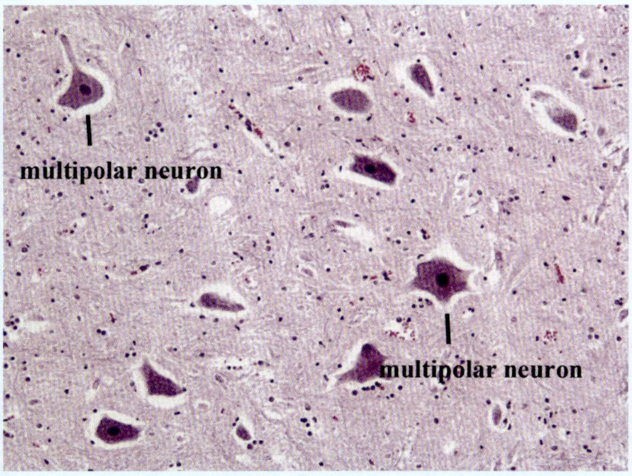

Fig. 25 Multipolar neuron (10×10)

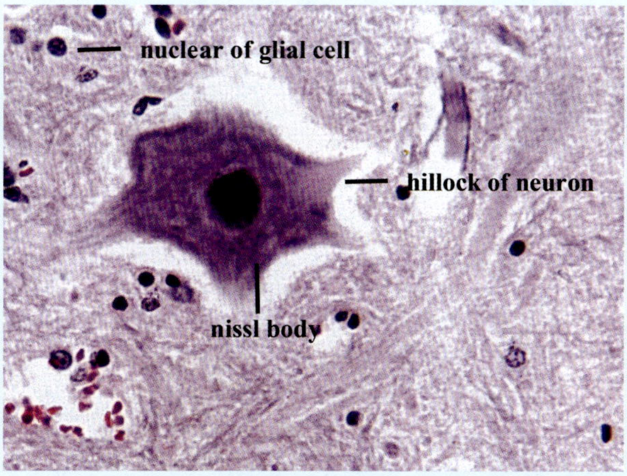

Fig. 26 Multipolar neuron (10×40)

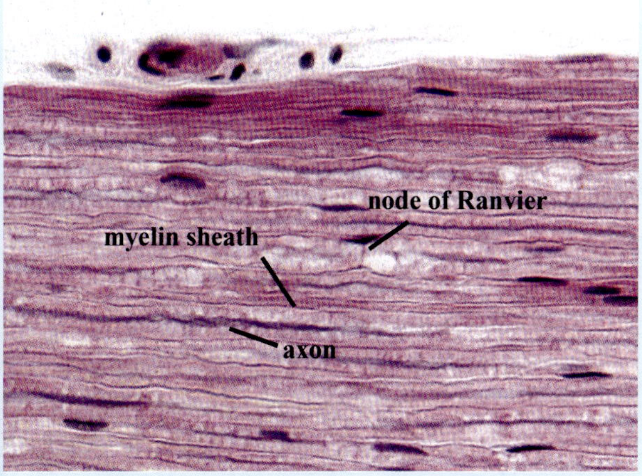

Fig. 27 Myelinated nerve fiber (10×40)

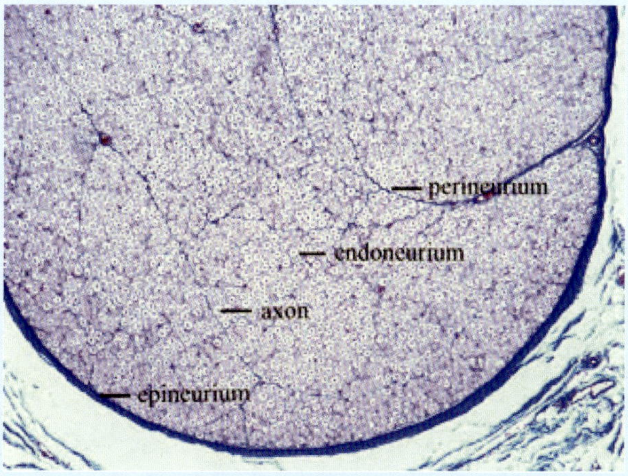

Fig. 28 Myelinated nerve fiber (10×4)

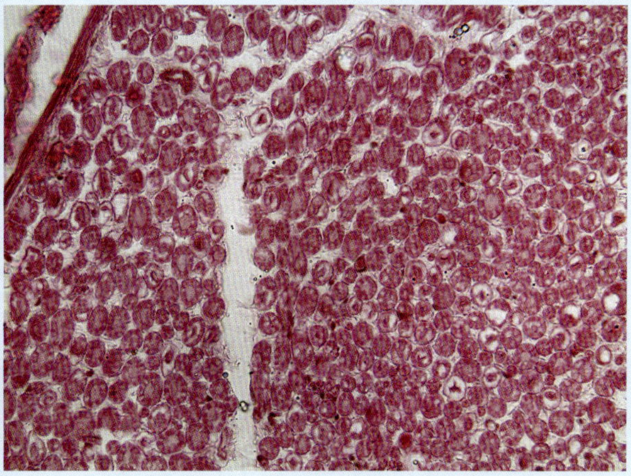

Fig. 29 Myelinated nerve fiber (10×10)

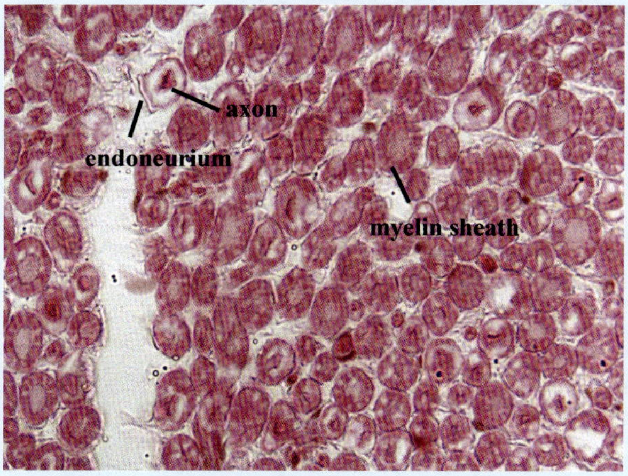

Fig. 30 Myelinated nerve fiber (10×40)

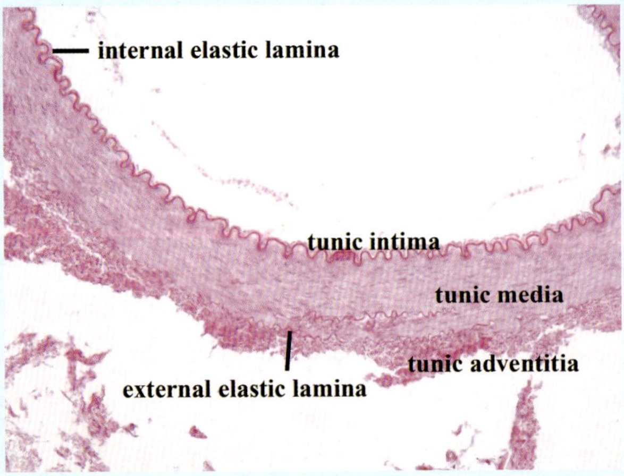

Fig. 31 Medium artery (10×10)

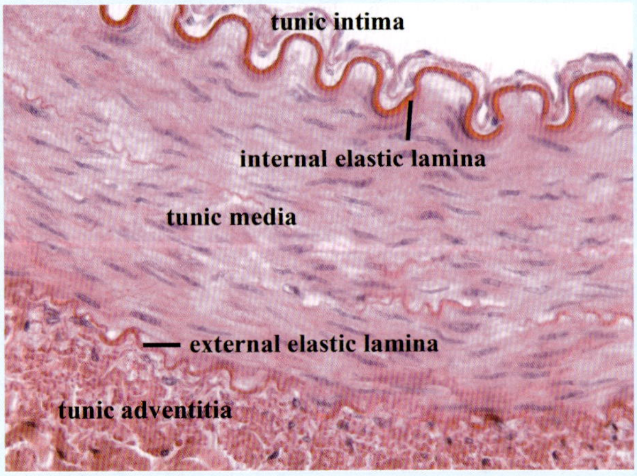

Fig. 32 Medium artery (10×40)

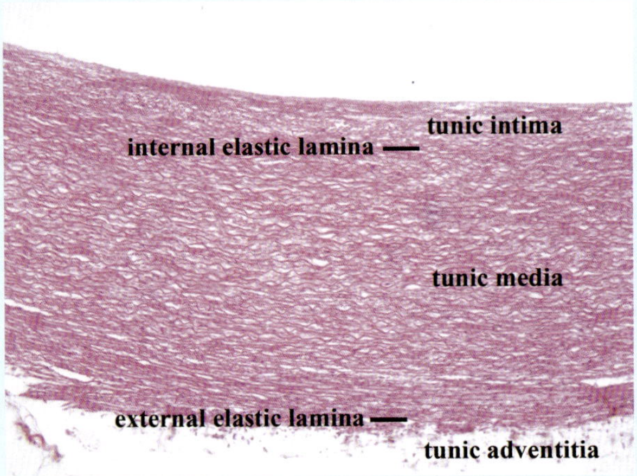

Fig. 33 Large artery (10×10)

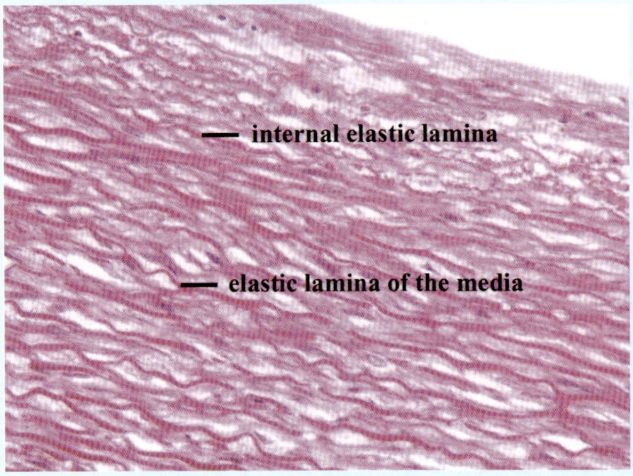

Fig. 34 Large artery (10×40)

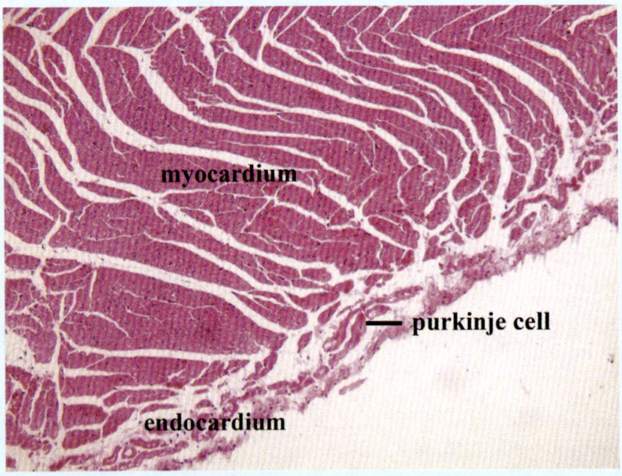

Fig. 35 Heart (10×10)

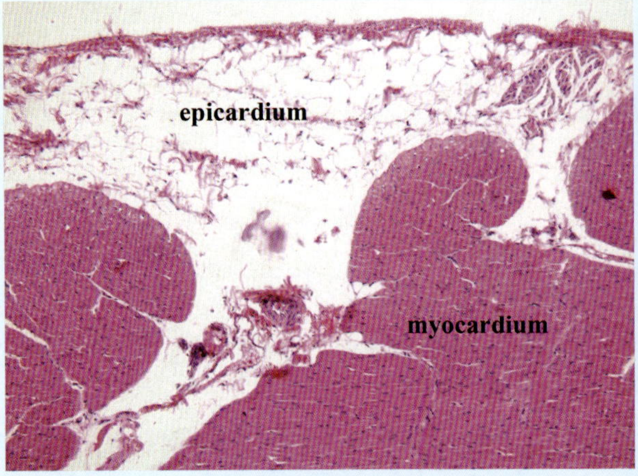

Fig. 36 Heart (10×10)

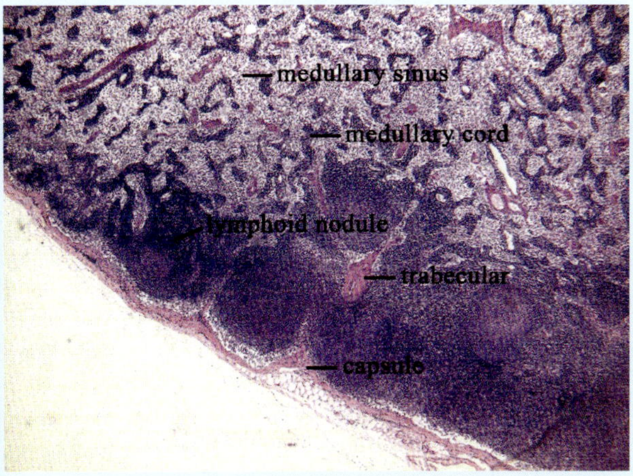

Fig. 37 Lymph node (10×4)

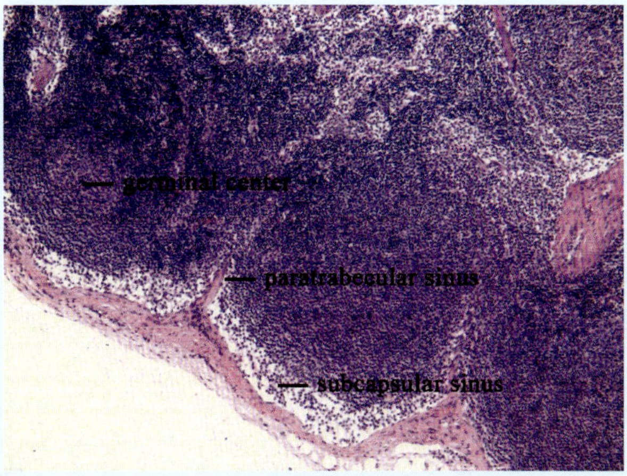

Fig. 38 Lymph node (10× 10)

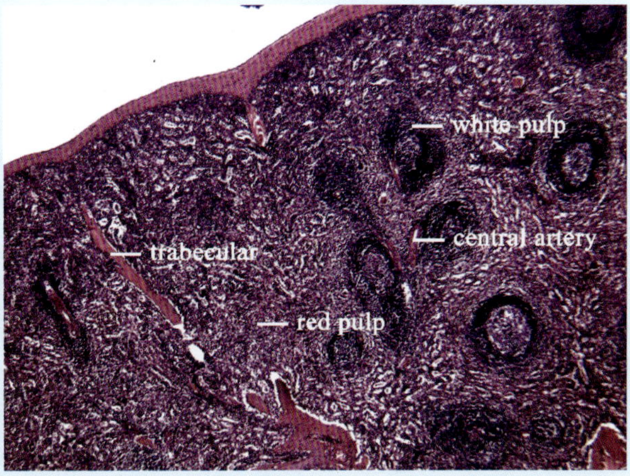

Fig. 39 Spleen (10×4)

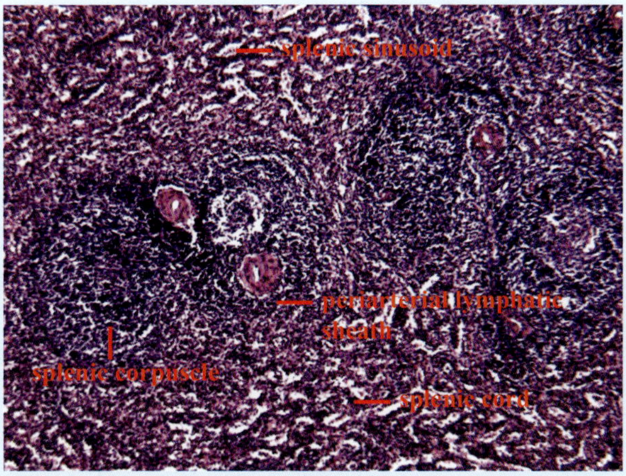

Fig. 40 Spleen (10×10)

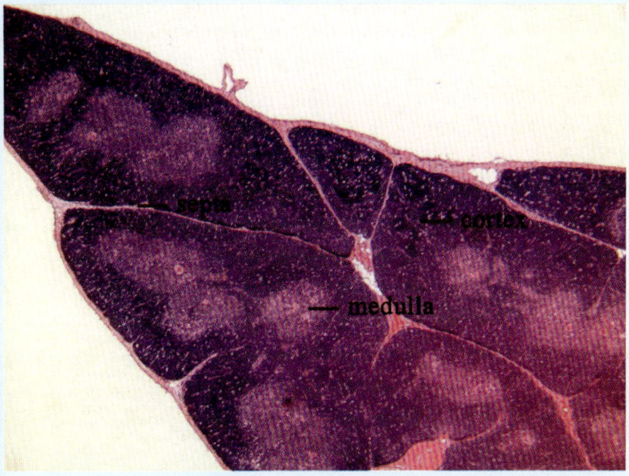

Fig. 41 Thymus (10×4)

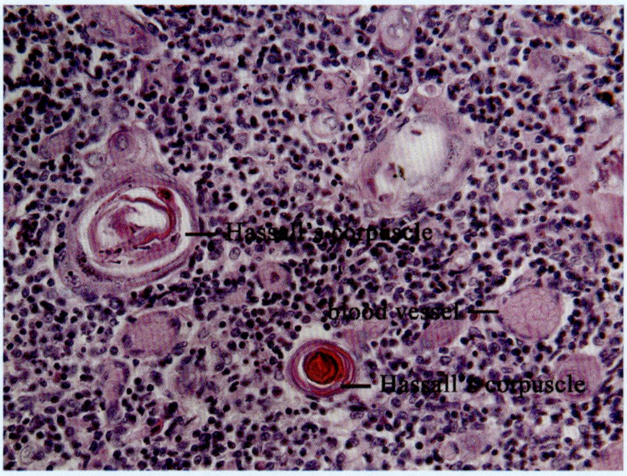

Fig. 42 Thymus (10×40)

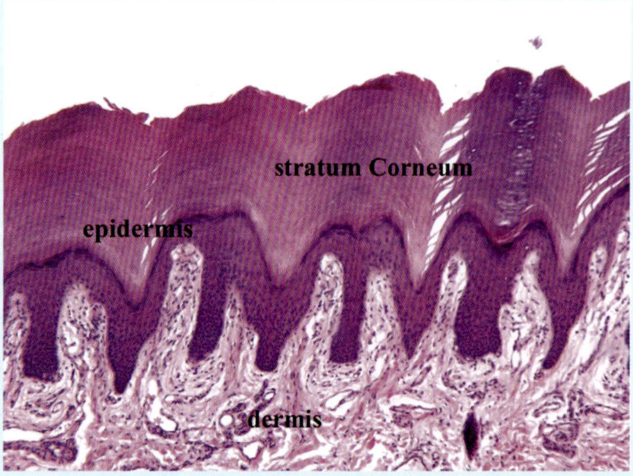

Fig. 43 Skin (palm) (10×10)

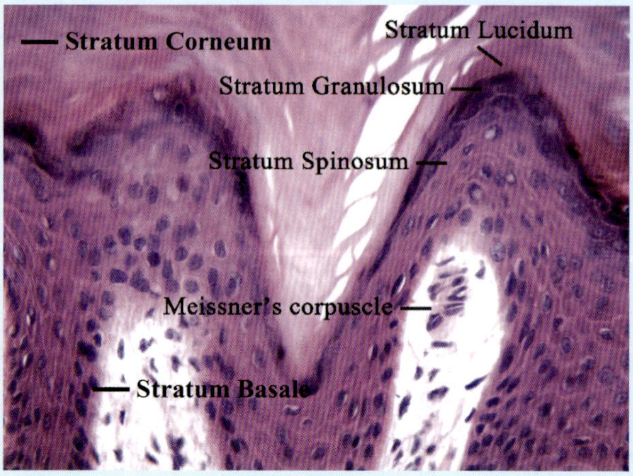

Fig. 44 Skin (palm) (10×40)

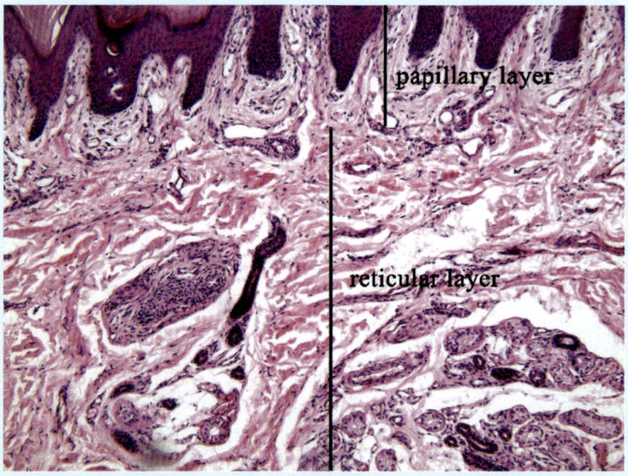

Fig. 45 Skin (palm) (10×10)

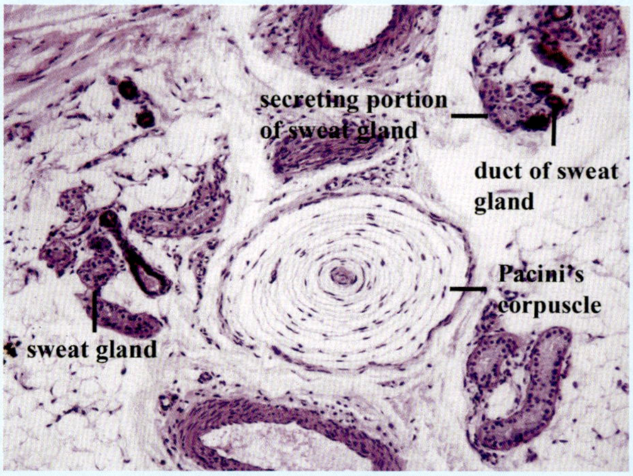

Fig. 46 Skin (palm) (10×40)

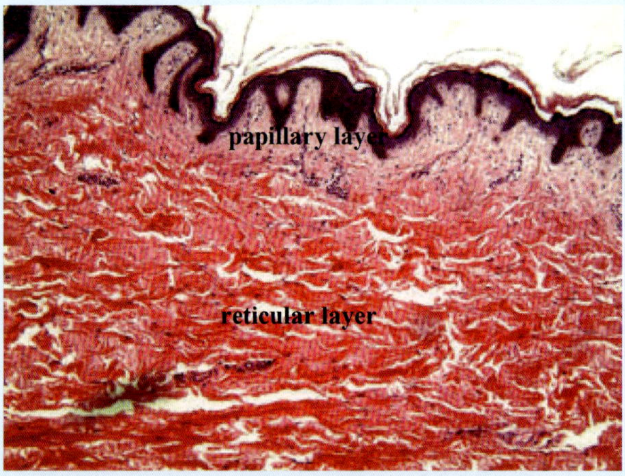

Fig. 47 Skin (body) (10×10)

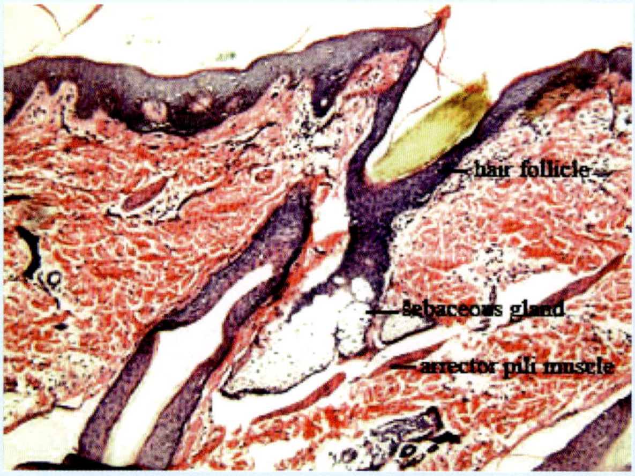

Fig. 48 Skin (head) (10×10)

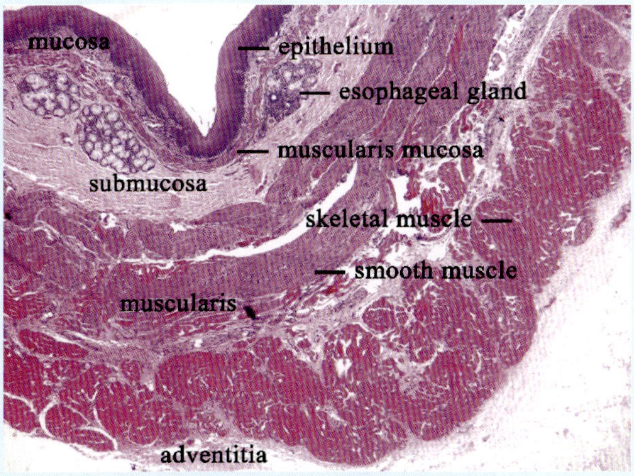

Fig. 49 Esophagus (10×4)

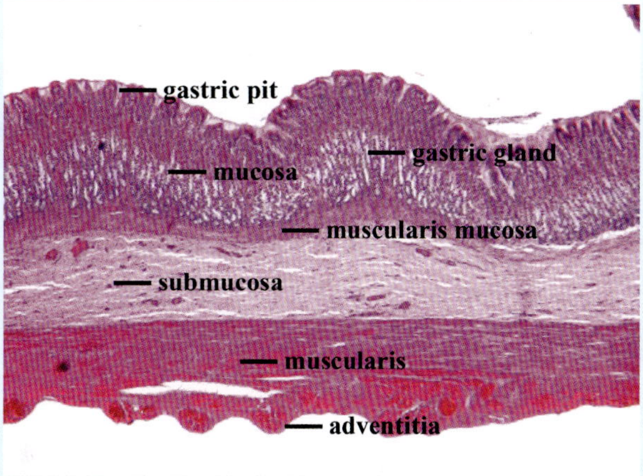

Fig. 50 Stomach (10×4)

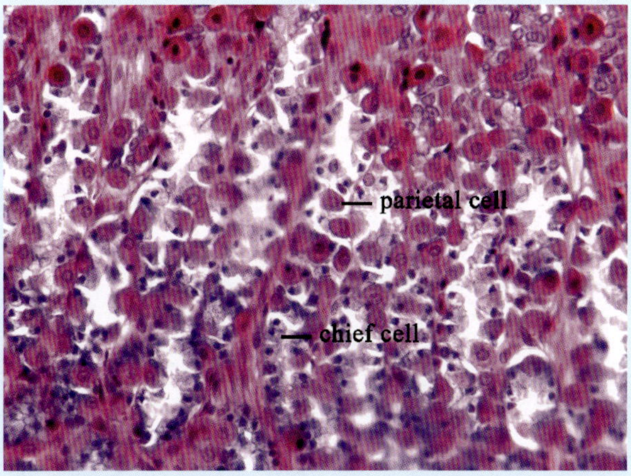

Fig. 51 Stomach (10×40)

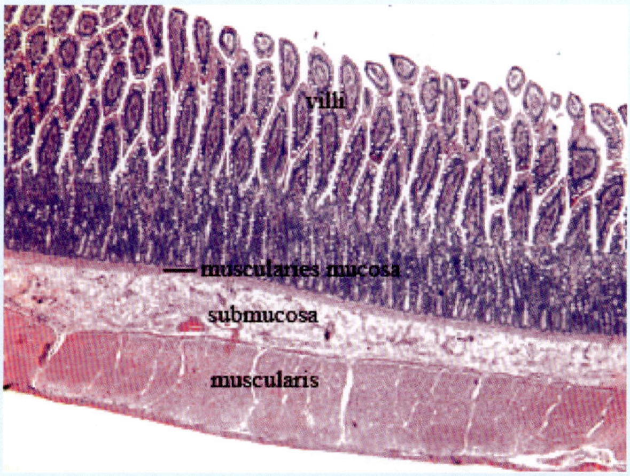

Fig. 52 Jejunum (10×4)

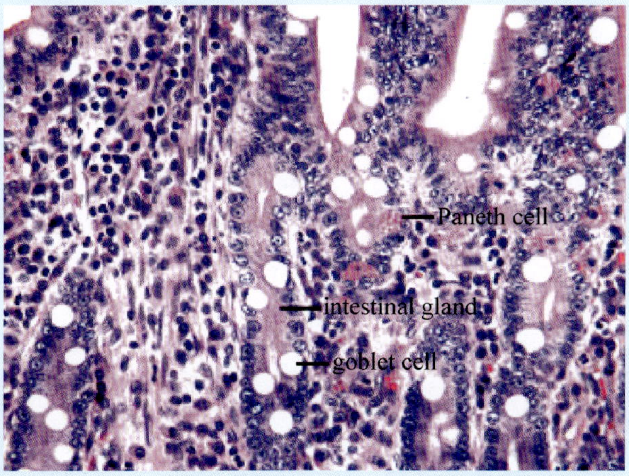

Fig. 53 Jejunum (10×40)

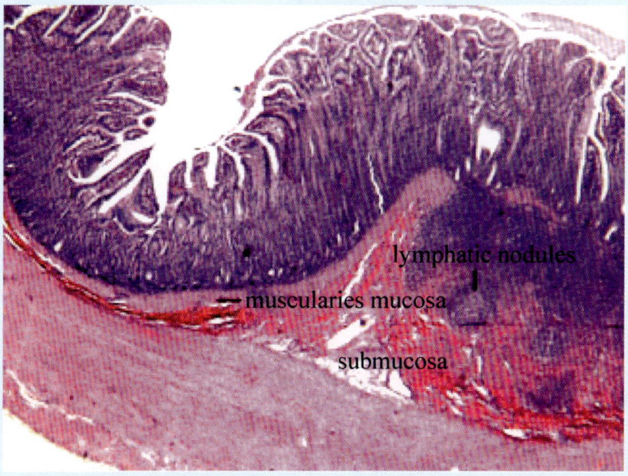

Fig. 54 Ileum (10×4)

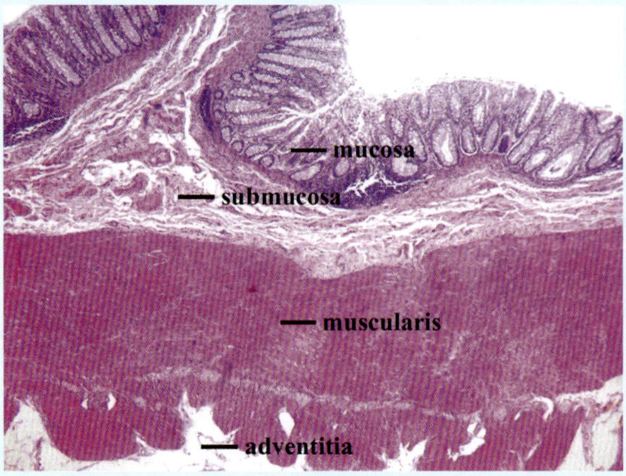

Fig. 55 Colon (10×4)

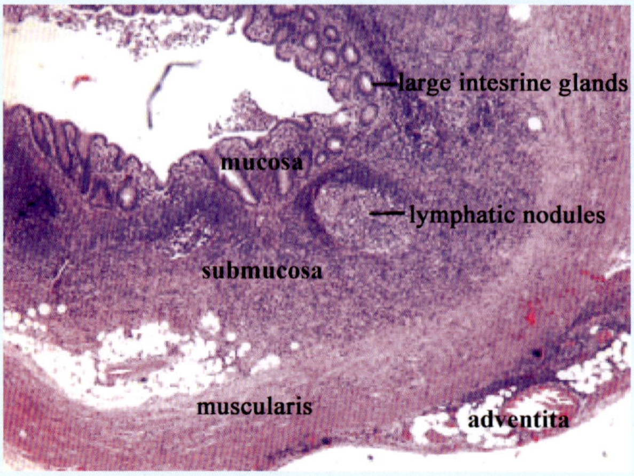

Fig. 56 Colon (10×40)

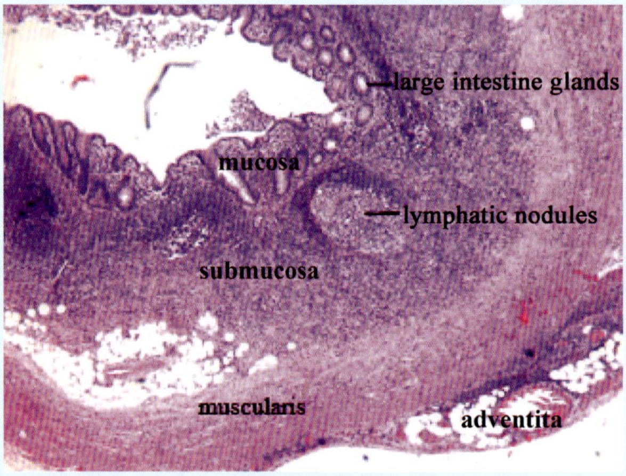

Fig. 57 Appendix (10×4)

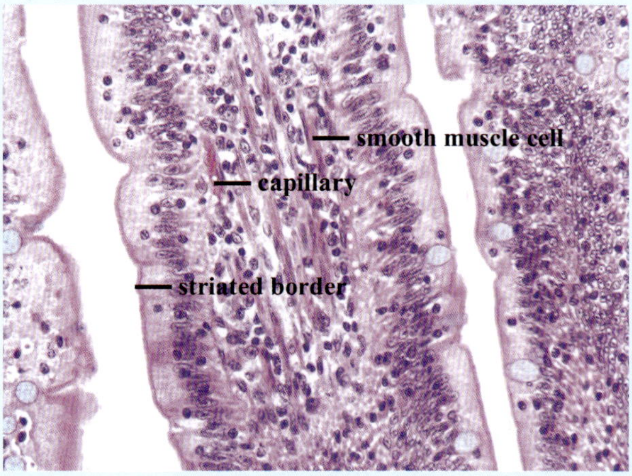

Fig. 58 Villus (10×40)

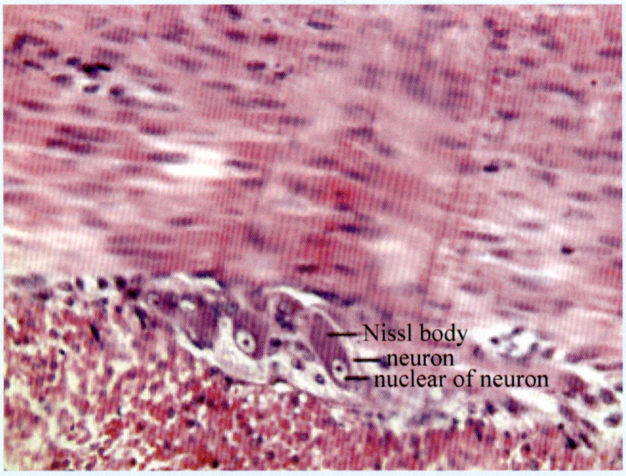

Fig. 59 Myenteric nerve plexus (10×40)

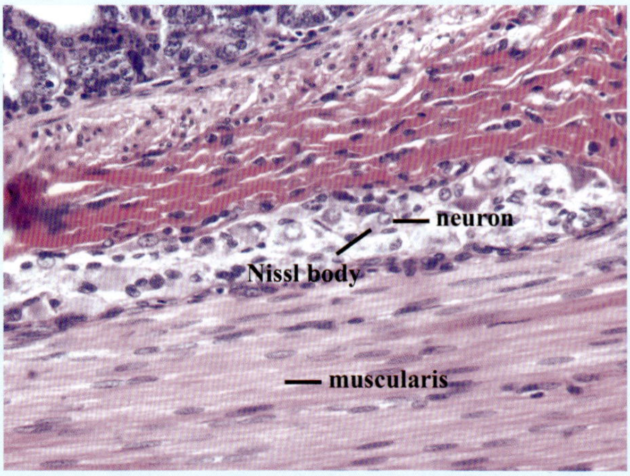

Fig. 60 Submucosal plexus (10×40)

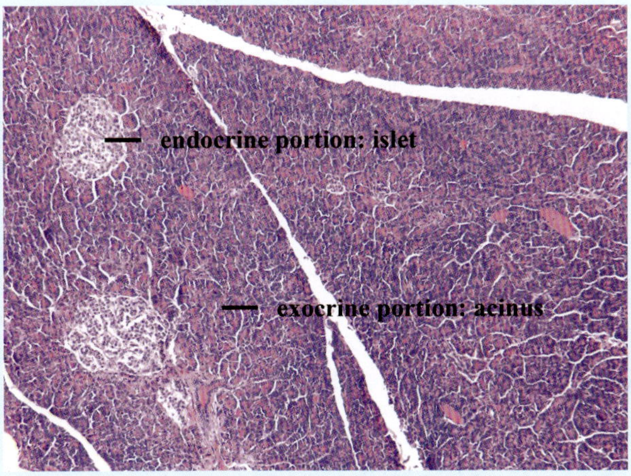

Fig. 61 Pancreas (10×10)

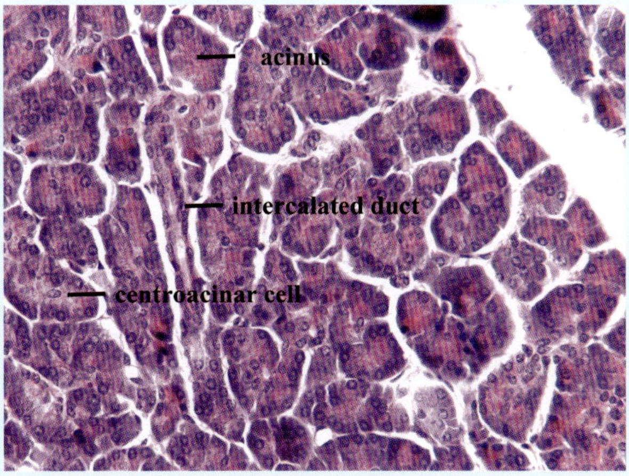

Fig. 62 Pancreas (10×40)

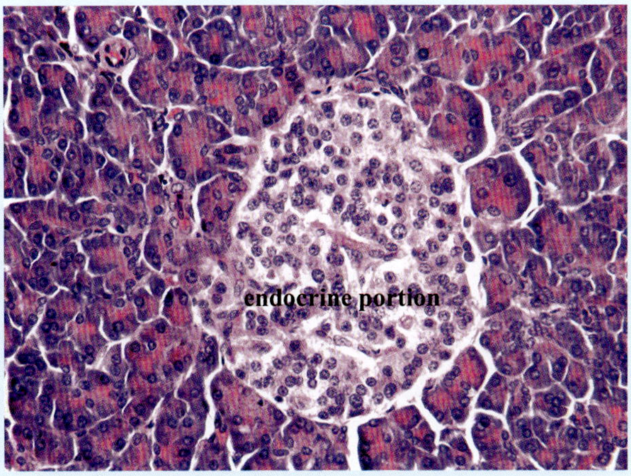

Fig. 63 Pancreas (10×40)

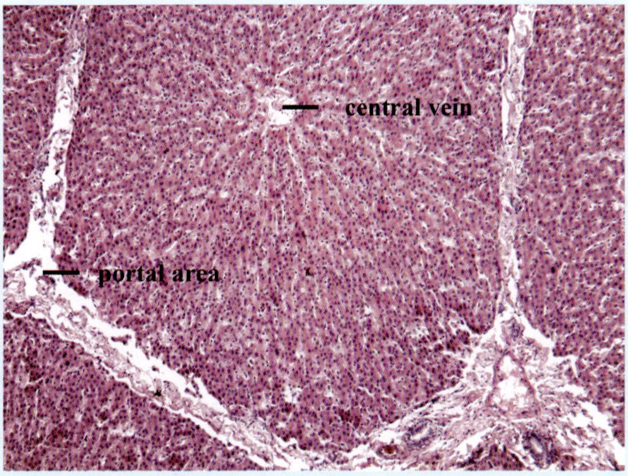

Fig. 64 Liver (Pig) (10×10)

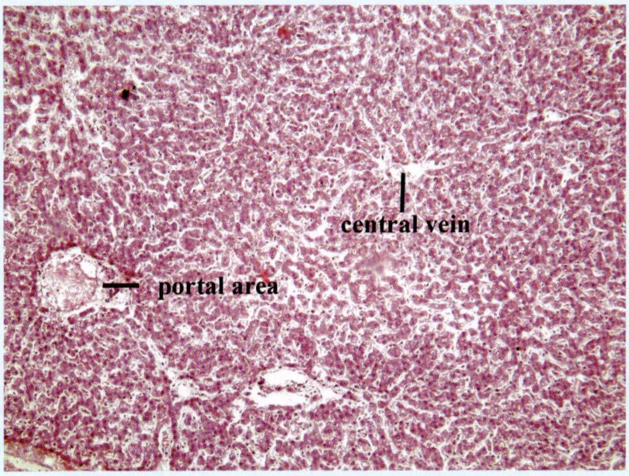

Fig. 65 Liver (Human) (10×10)

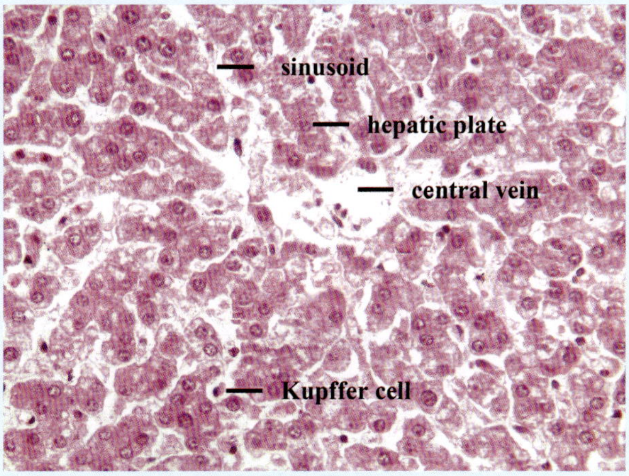

Fig. 66 Liver (Human) (10×40)

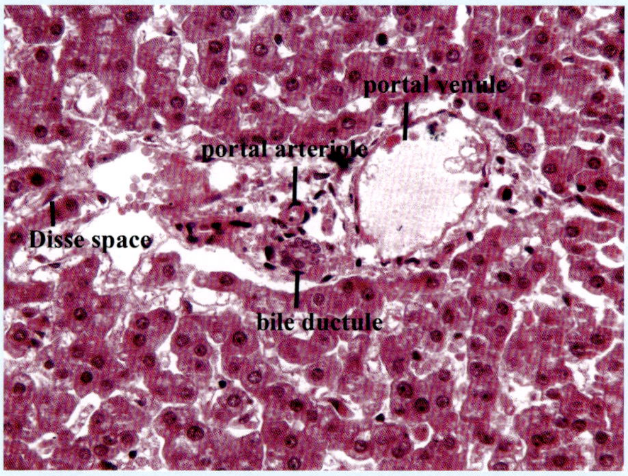

Fig. 67 Liver (Human) (10×40)

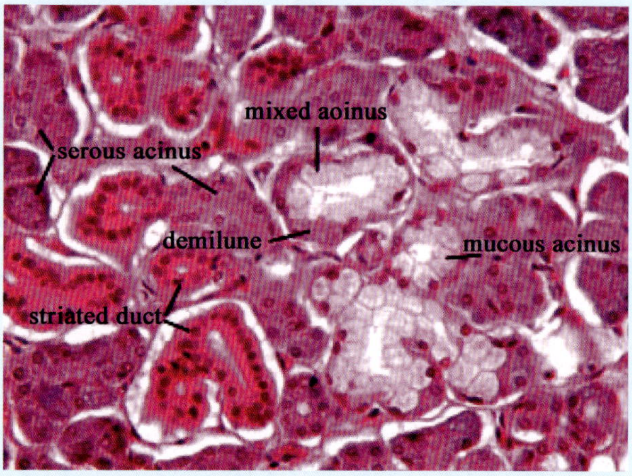

Fig. 68 Submandibular gland (10×40)

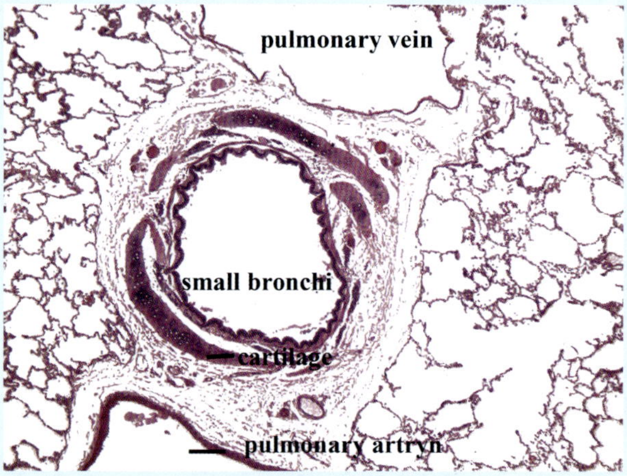

Fig. 69 Lung (10×10)

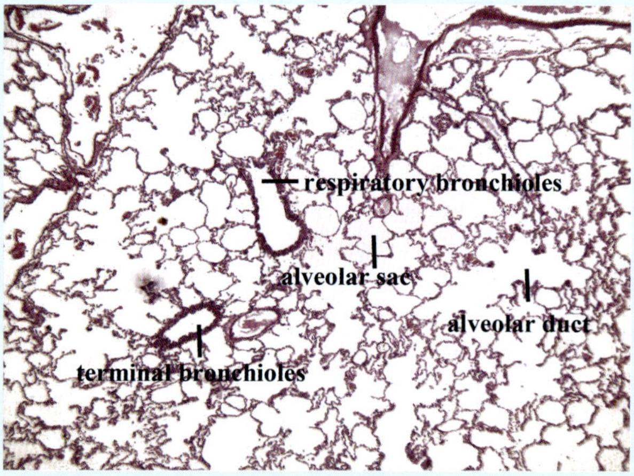

Fig. 70 Lung (10×4)

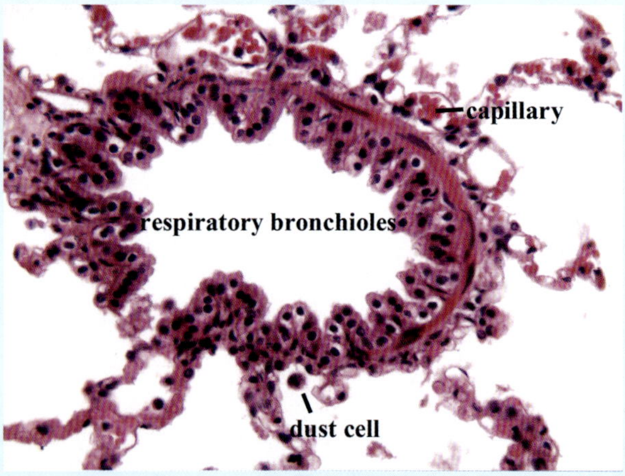

Fig. 71 Lung (10×40)

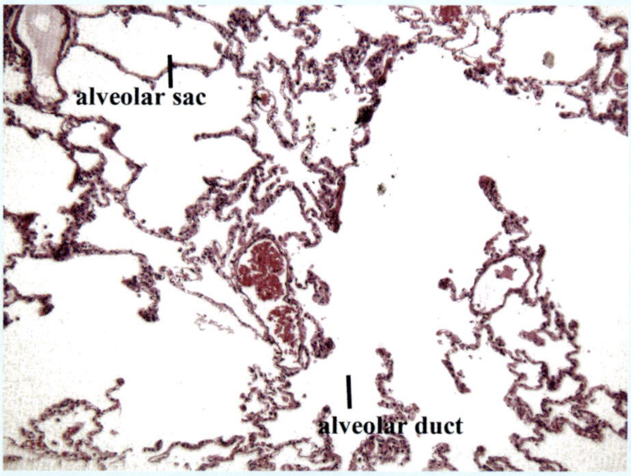

Fig. 72 Lung (10×10)

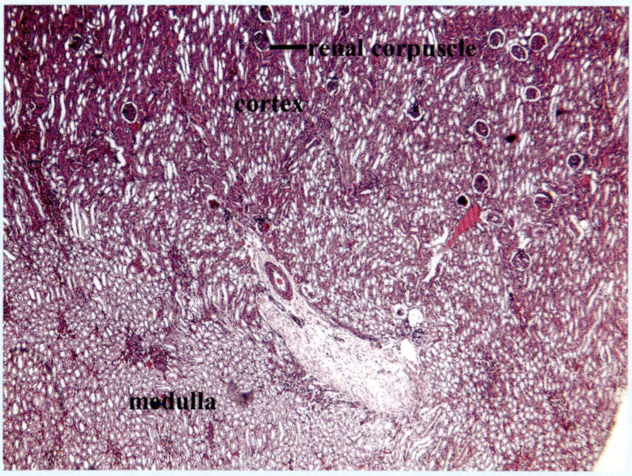

Fig. 73 Kindey (10×10)

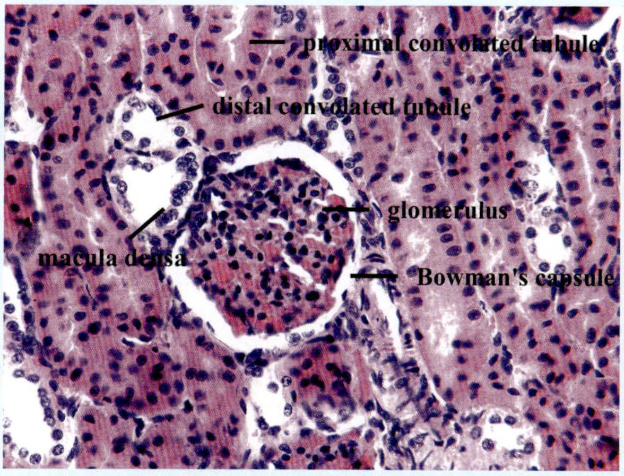

Fig. 74 Kindey (10×40)

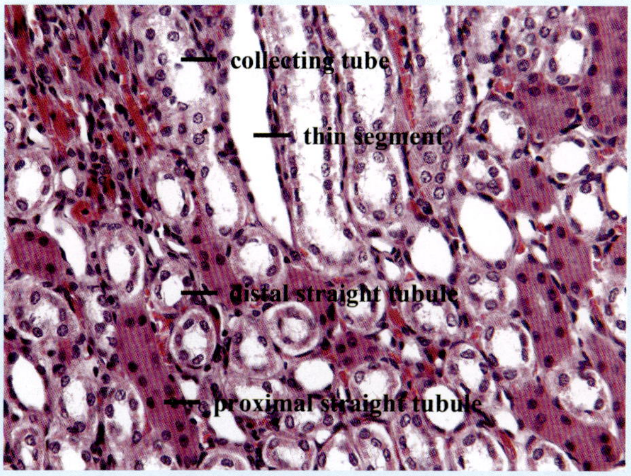

Fig. 75 Kindey (10×40)

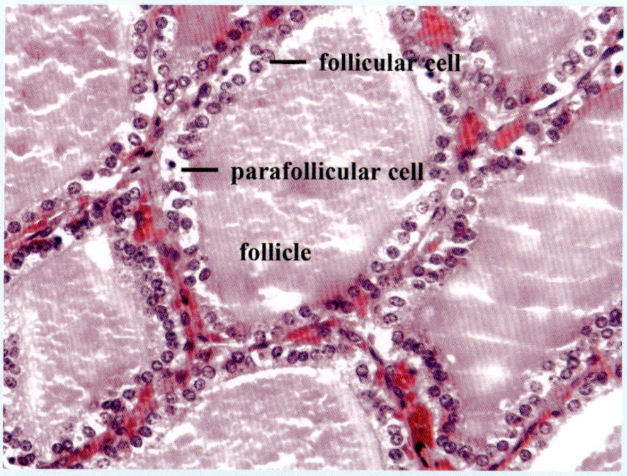

Fig. 76 Thyroid gland (10×40)

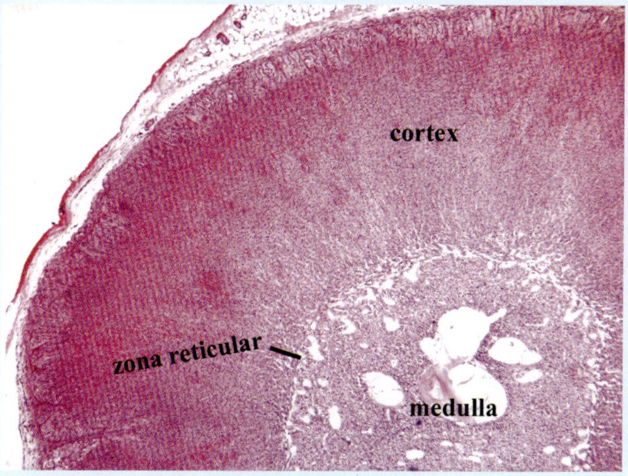

Fig. 77 Adrenal gland (10×4)

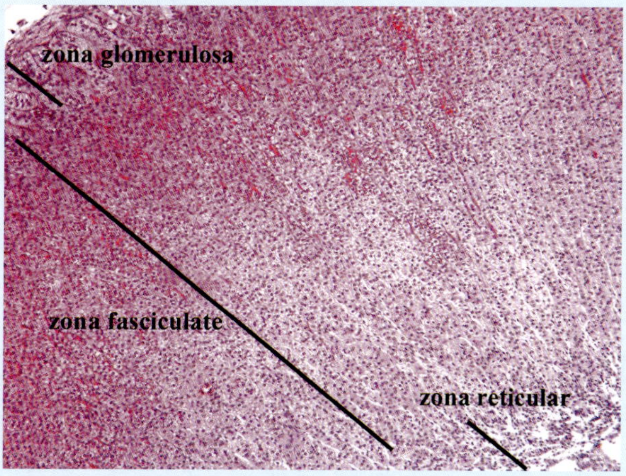

Fig. 78 Adrenal gland (10×10)

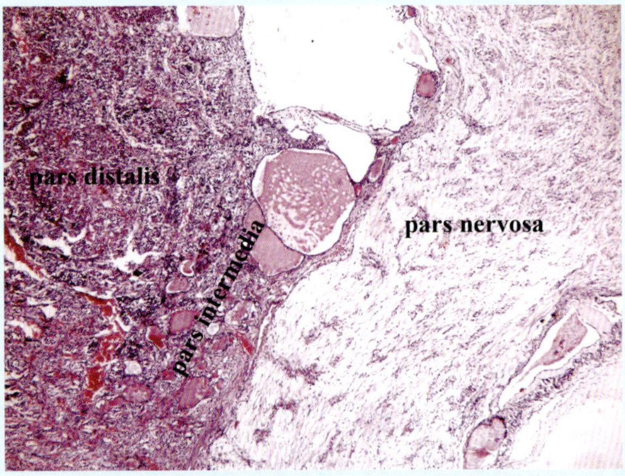

Fig. 79 Hypophysis (10×10)

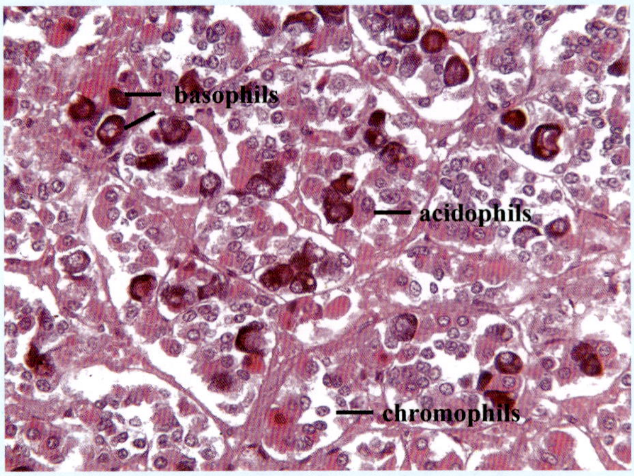

Fig. 80 Hypophysis (10×40)

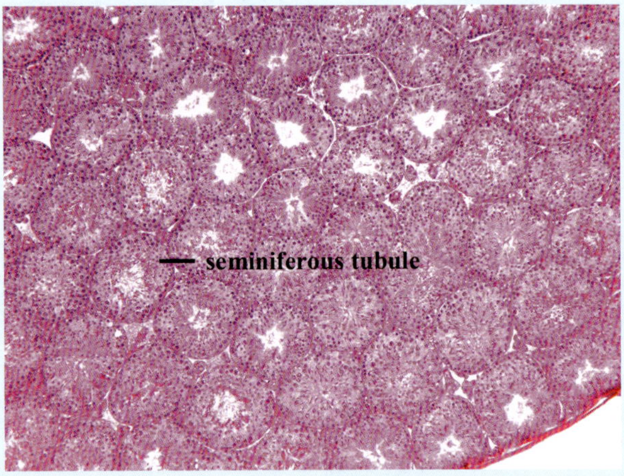

Fig. 81 Testis (10×10)

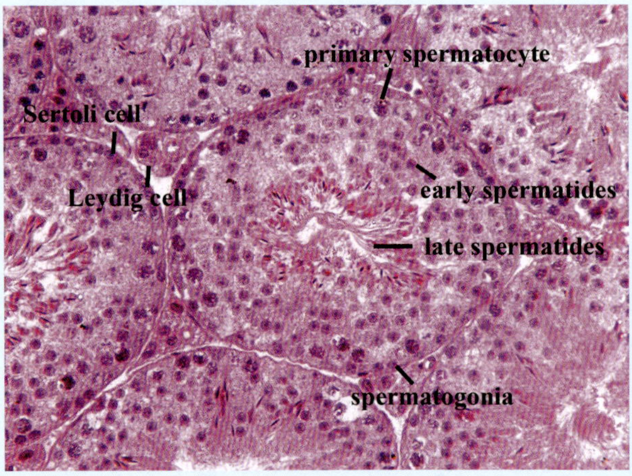

Fig. 82 Testis (10×40)

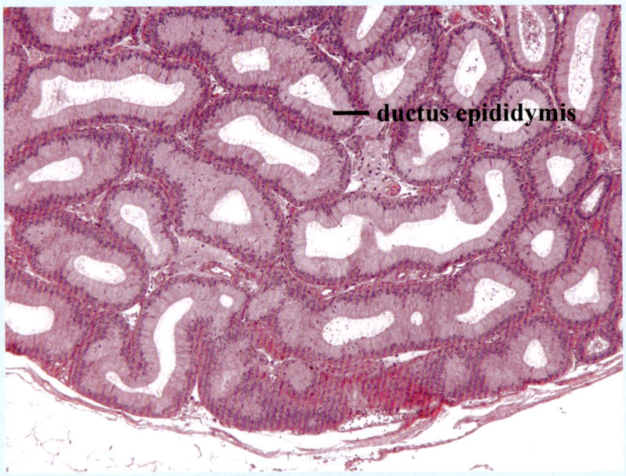

Fig. 83 Epididymis (10×10)

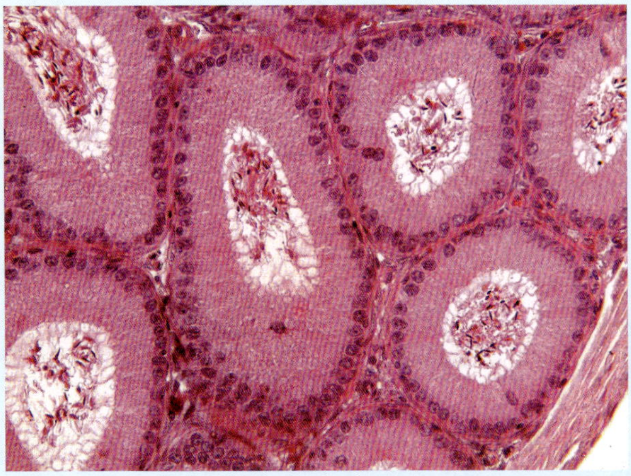

Fig. 84 Epididymis (10×40)

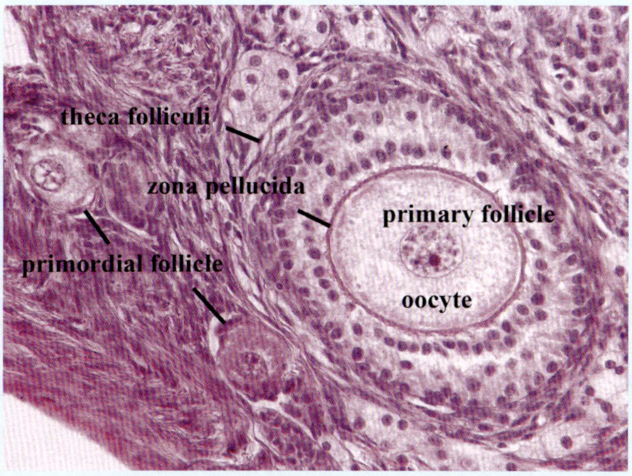

Fig. 85 Ovary (10×40)

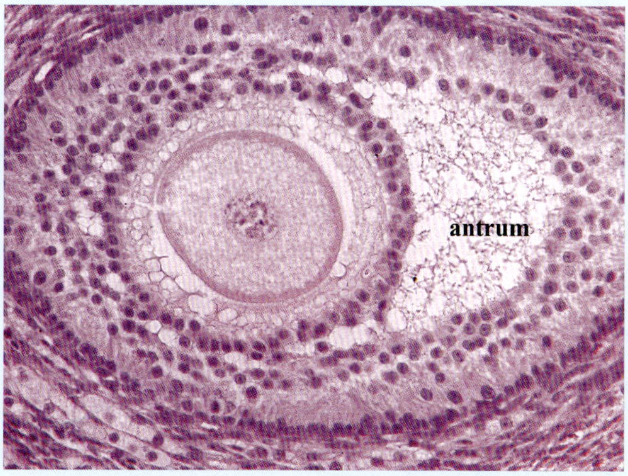

Fig. 86 Ovary (10×40)

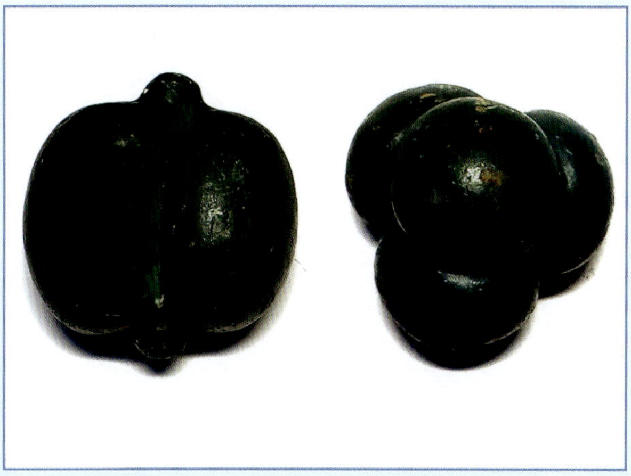

Fig. 87 Two-cell stage and four-cell stage

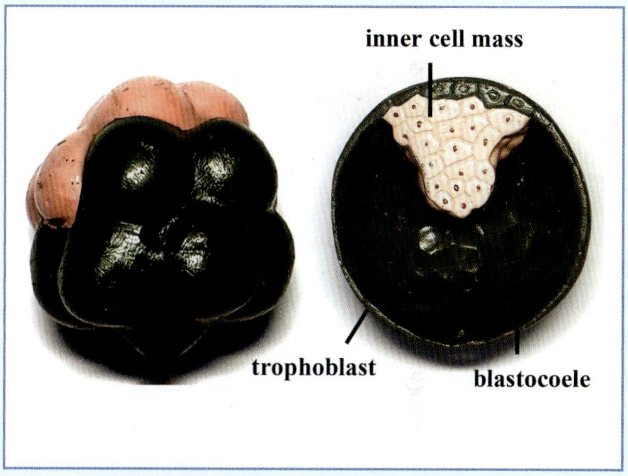

Fig. 88 Morula and blastocyst

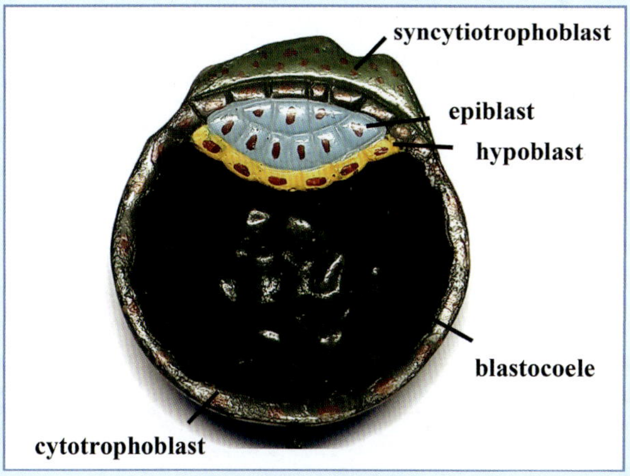

Fig. 89 Blastocyst

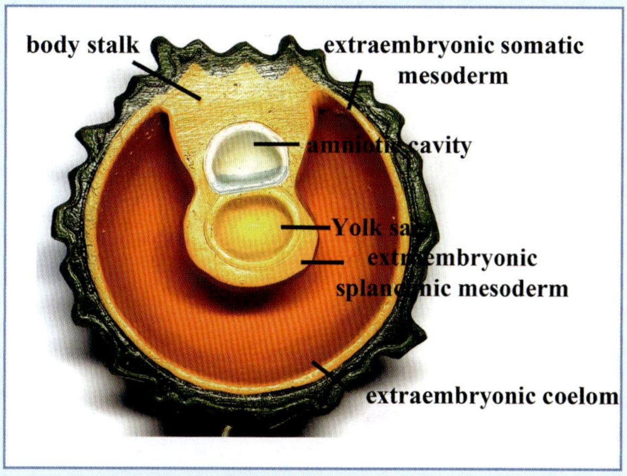

Fig. 90 Formation of bilaminar germ disc

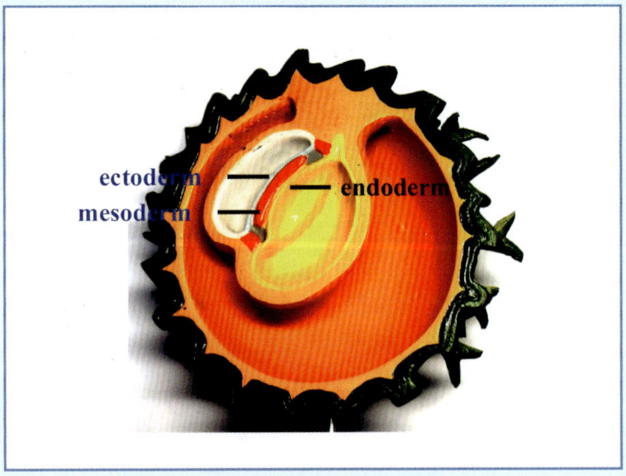

Fig. 91 Formation of trilaminar germ disc

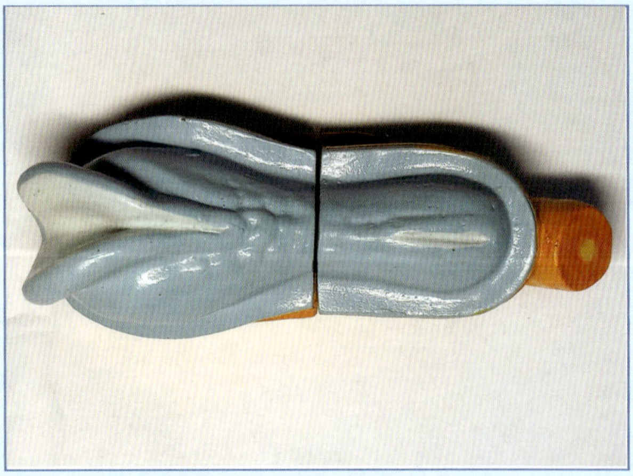

Fig. 92 Formation of neural tube

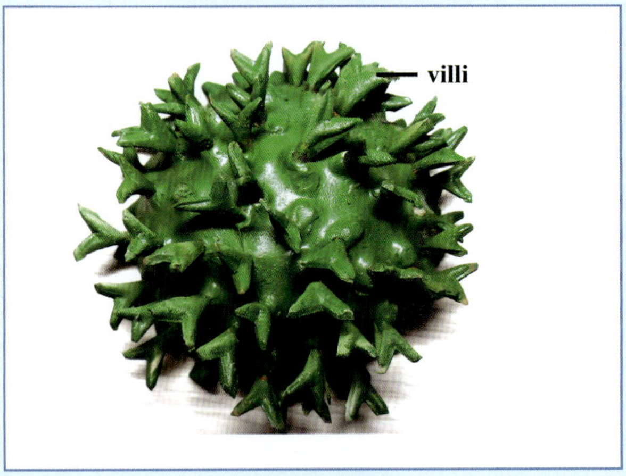

Fig. 93 Villi

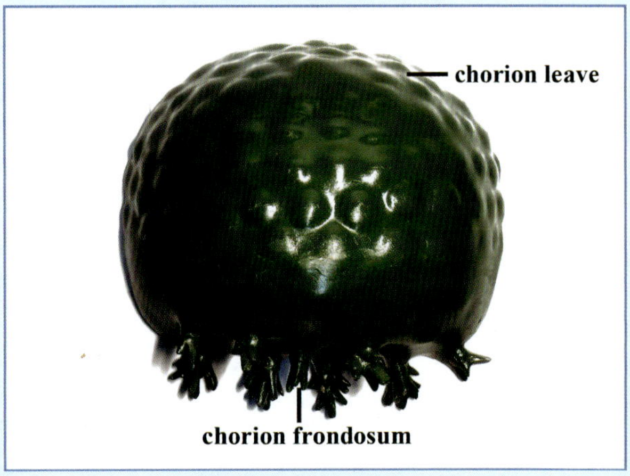

Fig. 94 Chorion

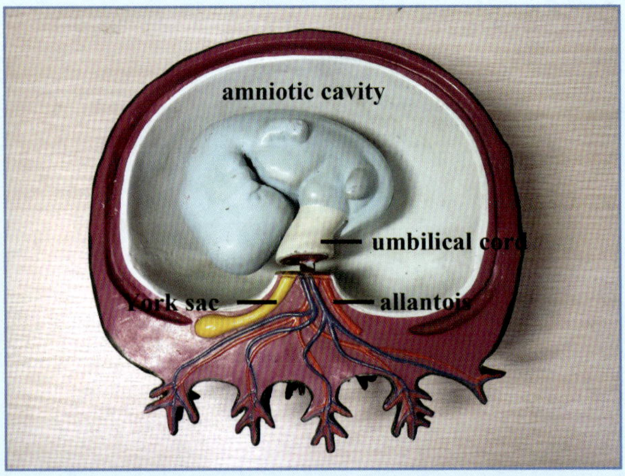

Fig. 95 Fetal membrane

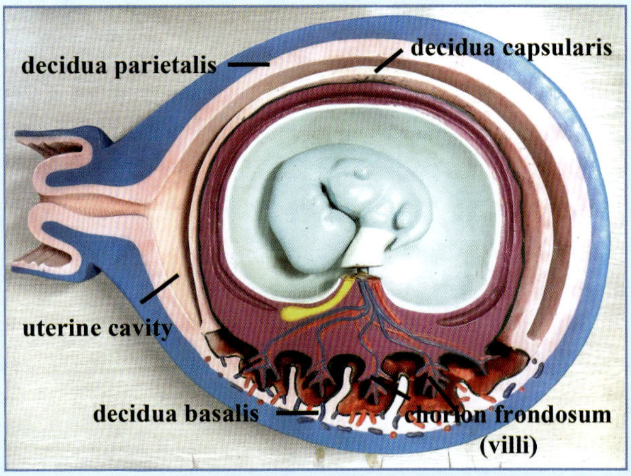

Fig. 96 Pregnant uterus